THE LUO COLLATERALS

by the same author

The Divergent Channels – Jing Bie
A Handbook of Clinical Practice and Five Shen Nei Dan Inner Meditation
ISBN 978 1 84819 189 1
eISBN 978 0 85701 150 3

Eight Extraordinary Channels – Qi Jing Ba Mai
A Handbook for Clinical Practice and Nei Dan Inner Meditation
ISBN 978 1 84819 148 8
eISBN 978 0 85701 137 4

I Ching Acupuncture – The Balance Method
Clinical Applications of the Ba Gua and I Ching
ISBN 978 1 84819 074 0
eISBN 978 0 85701 064 3

of related interest

Heavenly Stems and Earthly Branches – TianGan DiZhi
The Heart of Chinese Wisdom Traditions
Master Zhongxian Wu and Dr. Karin Taylor Wu
Foreword by Fei BingXun
ISBN 978 1 84819 151 8
eISBN 978 0 85701 158 9

Developing Internal Energy for Effective Acupuncture Practice
Zhan Zhuang, Yi Qi Gong and the Art of Painless Needle Insertion
Ioannis Solos
ISBN 978 1 84819 183 9
eISBN 978 0 85701 144 2

Acupuncture and Chinese Medicine
Roots of Modern Practice
Charles Buck
ISBN 978 1 84819 159 4
eISBN 978 0 85701 133 6

THE LUO COLLATERALS

A Handbook for Clinical Practice and Treating Emotions and the Shen and The Six Healing Sounds

DR. DAVID TWICKEN, DOM, L.AC.

SINGING DRAGON
LONDON AND PHILADELPHIA

First published in 2015
by Singing Dragon
an imprint of Jessica Kingsley Publishers
73 Collier Street
London N1 9BE, UK
and
400 Market Street, Suite 400
Philadelphia, PA 19106, USA

www.singingdragon.com

Library of Congress Cataloging in Publication Data
Twicken, David, author.
The luo collaterals : a handbook of clinical practice and treating emotions and the shen and the six healing sounds / Dr. David Twicken.
p. ; cm
Includes bibliographical references and index.
ISBN 978-1-84819-230-0 (alk. paper)
I. Title.
[DNLM: 1. Meridians--Case Reports. 2. Acupuncture Therapy--Case Reports. 3. Medicine, Chinese Traditional--Case Reports. 4. Qigong--Case Reports. WB 369.5.M5]
RM184.5
615.8'92--dc23

2015014567

British Library Cataloguing in Publication Data
A CIP catalogue record for this book is available from the British Library

ISBN 978 1 84819 230 0
eISBN 978 0 85701 219 7

Printed and bound in Great Britain

FSC
www.fsc.org
MIX
Paper from responsible sources
FSC® C013604

CONTENTS

DISCLAIMER

The information in this book is based on the author's knowledge and personal experience. This information is presented for educational purposes to assist the reader in expanding his or her knowledge of Chinese philosophy and Chinese medicine. The techniques and practices are to be used at the reader's own discretion and liability. The author is not responsible in any manner whatsoever for any physical injury that may occur by following instructions in this book. Consult a licensed physician for any health condition.

ACKNOWLEDGMENTS

I would like to give a special thank you to Master Mantak Chia for sharing qi gong, internal alchemy and Taoism with compassion, respect and love.

Thank you, Yitian Ni and Complementary Medicine Press, for the luo collaterals illustrations in Chapter 2.

Thank you, Dr. Lorraine Wilcox, Ph.D., L.Ac., and the Chinese Medicine Database, for permission to use material from Volume V of the *Zhen Jiu Da Cheng* (*The Great Compendium of Acupuncture and Moxibustion*).

Thank you, my good friend Gregory E. Leblanc, L.Ac., and my colleague Dr. Fritz Hudnut, DAOM, L.Ac., for your editorial contributions.

Thank you, Jacques MoraMarco, OMD, L.Ac., for your contributions about the history of the French practitioners George Soulié de Morant and Dr. Albert Chamfrault.

A special thank you to Dr. Lorraine Wilcox, Ph.D., L.Ac., for providing me with professional-level translations and interpretations from the *Ling Shu*, *Su Wen* and the *Zhen Jiu Da Cheng*. I am very grateful for your generosity of time and your expert knowledge.

Thank you, Jessica Kingsley and your excellent team at Singing Dragon, for all your work in publishing this book.

AUTHOR NOTE

The Luo Collaterals: A Handbook for Clinical Practice and Treating Emotions and the Shen and The Six Healing Sounds is the fourth in a series of books on Chinese medicine and the Taoist arts. The luo collaterals are part of the channel system presented in the Han dynasty classics, the *Su Wen* and the *Ling Shu*. These collaterals play an important role in the clinical applications of acupuncture. This book includes a journey along the path left by the ancient practitioners of Chinese medicine and Taoist healing. Understanding the origins of the channel system is essential in evaluating and applying modern interpretations and clinical applications. Our journey ranges from the Han dynasty to the twenty-first century; main changes about the luo collaterals are identified and evaluated. This book includes a detailed history of the *window of the sky points* and a Taoist and Chinese medical understanding of emotions, the five shen and the Shen; this information is the basis for clinical practice. This book also includes a comprehensive presentation of the six healing sounds of qi gong and how they treat emotions, and the five shen.

My books *I Ching Acupuncture—The Balance Method*; *Eight Extraordinary Channels—Qi Jing Ba Mai*; *The Divergent Channels—Jing Bie*; and *The Luo Collaterals* provide a framework for clinical practice. Understanding and applying all the channel systems in clinical practice is the insight of the ancient practitioners of Chinese medicine. In my experience as a practitioner and clinical supervisor at Chinese medical schools, including all the channels in clinical practice significantly increases clinical efficacy. I hope this book assists you in applying the luo mai in clinical practice.

INTRODUCTION

Two thousand years ago the Chinese shifted from the belief that supernatural intervention was the cause of illness. The shift led to the development of one of the oldest systems of holistic medicine. Chinese medicine is a deep and wide healing system that is rooted in the understanding that humanity is part of its environment. The ancient Chinese people deeply observed the influences of the stars, the planets and the seasons on humanity. These people perceived the resonance between nature and humanity. They deeply studied astronomy and mapped out the celestial bodies; this was the cosmic map. They turned their focus inward and perceived the energy fields and the physical structures within the human body; this was the inner map. The inner map is a magnificent, detailed and comprehensive guide to the structure and functioning of the human body. The inner map is presented in the early Chinese medical classic texts, the *Su Wen* and the *Ling Shu*. This map contains the following acupuncture channel system:

- cutaneous channels
- muscle (sinew) channels
- connecting (luo) collaterals
- primary (main) channels
- divergent (separate) channels
- eight extraordinary channels.

The inner map of the human body is the terrain for the interaction of substances within the body. The following passage is from the *Su Wen*,

Chapter 27, "Pathogens." It captures this insight and provides the foundation for diagnosis.

> A well-rounded physician must have a certain set of principles in medicine and he/she must also observe the changes in nature. For example, in heavens there are changes in the positions of the sun, the moon with its waxing and waning, and the constellations. On the earth there are rivers, tributaries, and oceans. In human beings there are the channels and luo mai. These influence each other. When the weather warms, the flow of waters in the rivers becomes calm and easy. When the weather is cold, the flow of water stagnates. When the weather is excessively hot, however, the waters in the rivers become abundant, and flooding results. If the storms begin, further disasters occur. Similarly, an external pathogen invades the body. Cold causes the channels and collateral blood and qi to stagnate. Heat will cause blood to flow very freely and rapidly. Excessive heat will cause the channels and luo mai to swell.[1]

This *Su Wen* passage expresses how patterns and interactions in nature were perceived as mirrors of the interactions in the human body. The early contributors of Chinese philosophy and medicine saw a deep parallel between nature and humanity. They described their insights in classic medical texts. Two common pathogenic factors presented in the classic medical texts are heat and cold. These pathogenic factors are the main pathogens that influence the luo mai (connecting collaterals). In the acupuncture channel system the luo mai are located at the superficial level of the body. If pathogens in the luo mai are not effectively treated they can be transferred deeper into the channel system and to the internal organs. Additionally, pathogens in the luo mai can block and stagnate the flow of qi and blood in their collaterals and throughout the body. Treating the luo mai is an essential aspect of Chinese medicine and a main treatment in the practice of acupuncture.

The luo mai are primarily presented in the *Ling Shu,* Chapter 10, "The Main Channels." The luo mai are also presented in the following *Su Wen* chapters: Chapter 21, "Meridian Pathology and Correspondences;" Chapter 24, "Channel Constituents and Acupuncture Techniques;" Chapter 39, "Differentiation of Pain;" Chapter 56, "Dermatomes of the Channels;"

Chapter 57, "Channels and Collaterals;" Chapter 58, "Acupuncture Points;" Chapter 62, "Regulation of the Channels;" and Chapter 63, "Acupuncturing the Superficial Luo." The luo mai are also called the luo collaterals and the linking collaterals.

The *Ling Shu* describes a few ways to distinguish the luo mai from the main channels.

1. The luo mai are visible. The main channels are invisible.
2. The pulse does not measure the condition of the luo mai. The pulse does measure conditions of the main channels.
3. The luo mai flow through small articulations—they do not flow through the main joints. The luo mai flow through alternate routes (the main and divergent channel pathways flow through large articulations) of entering and exiting in their channel system to eventually join in the skin.
4. The luo mai are outlets for pathogens. The traditional treatment is bloodletting, which releases the pathogen with the blood from the body. It is interesting that the oldest book on Chinese medicine, the Mawangdui medical texts, has two main treatments: lancet (bloodletting) and moxibustion. The luo mai may be part of the insight of the earliest practitioners of Chinese medicine.

The structure, function and treatments for the luo mai have changed from the time of the *Su Wen* and the *Ling Shu.* I will present *Su Wen* and *Ling Shu* theories and applications. During the Ming dynasty, and especially at the turn of the twentieth century when Chinese medicine went to Europe, new interpretations and clinical applications were presented. I will present a timeline of when these new applications were presented. The ideas that make up the basis of these new methods will be presented as well. I hope that this presentation will spark a deeper study of them and provide the practitioner with more choices for clinical treatment.

The theory and clinical applications of the luo mai can be split into two main groups. The first is from the *Ling Shu,* with support from the *Jia Yi Jing* (*The Systematic Classic of Acupuncture and Moxibustion*), and the *Su Wen.* If there is a conflict between the *Su Wen* and the *Ling Shu,* I will defer to the latter; it is the classic book on acupuncture. The second group includes non-classical theories and applications that were developed centuries after these classics. The most common practiced applications were introduced in more recent times. These methods include using the source and luo points to treat the main channels and the internal organs. This method is called the host–guest treatment (there are other versions of the host–guest method). Another method is using the luo points for treating psycho-emotional conditions. Dou Hanqing introduced a third method in 1196 AD. He presented the theory that four of the connecting points were the opening points (also called confluent, command and master points) of the eight extraordinary channels. And that the four connecting points were used to treat the eight extraordinary channels. This led to new functions of the luo points. George Soulié de Morant, Dr. Albert Chamfrault and Dr. Nguyen Van Nghi contributed to the development of modern applications of the luo collaterals and the luo points. Each of these applications will be evaluated in this book.

Pricking is a bloodletting method. The use of a lancet or other pricking device is part of the earliest Chinese medical practice. Pricking is a practice that can be a luo mai treatment or a bloodletting treatment, which is a Chinese medical treatment of its own. Pricking as part of a luo mai treatment, which pricks only the luo mai and the luo point, is the clinical application found in the *Ling Shu*. Having a clear understanding of the differences between the two is important. To learn about pricking throughout the body I recommend a fantastic book: *Pricking the Vessels: Blood Letting Therapy in Chinese Medicine* by Dr. Henry McCann (2014).

The Luo Collaterals: A Handbook for Clinical Practice and Treating Emotions and the Shen and The Six Healing Sounds includes a classical Chinese medical and Taoist understanding of the shen, the five shen and emotions. (How we differentiate the Shen from the five shen is explained on p.60.) The chapter on emotions demonstrates how emotions are formed from a Chinese and Taoist medical perspective. The chapter provides an essential link between the luo mai, luo points and points on the main channels for treating emotions, the five shen and the Shen.

Healing Sounds Qi Gong is one of the oldest and most effective treatments for emotions, the internal organs and the five shen. A comprehensive theory and practice of the healing sounds is presented in this book. I have practiced this qi gong for 30 years, and have taught it at Chinese medical schools for 20 years. It is simple to learn, fun to practice and a very effective qi gong.

The luo mai are an integral part of the acupuncture channel system; they can be used to access conditions in their collaterals. In this case, the pathogens are in the luo mai. The luo mai can also be combined in treatments with other channels to release pathogenic factors in the body. In this condition, the pathogen is moved out of a channel system/area of the body to the luo mai at the superficial layer of the body, and then released with a luo mai treatment. The luo mai make up a powerful channel system for clinical practice and are an essential aspect in the practice of acupuncture.

The theories and clinical applications of the luo mai have changed through the history of Chinese medicine. This book will trace the path left by the early *Su Wen* and *Ling Shu* practitioners, which will provide a framework for clinical practice. This framework includes a guide on how to use all the channel systems. Each channel system has specific functions. In my experience, being able to clinically apply all of the channels allows the practitioner to obtain the best clinical results. The *Ling Shu* and the *Su Wen* offer the original theories and clinical applications of the luo mai. These theories and applications will be presented first; other applications will follow. Studying the original theories and applications can provide practitioners with the flexibility to change the way they practice to meet changing conditions and environments. Having a comprehensive understanding of the acupuncture channel system provides the foundation to create unique treatments for each person. This is the essence of holistic healing and Chinese medicine.

CHAPTER 1

THE LUO MAI

The luo collaterals connect with the 365 points and correspond to the 365 days of the year. The function of the collaterals is to dispel the pathogen from the channels, and to promote the flow of the ying/nutritive and wei/defensive.[2]

The insights of the early writers and practitioners of Chinese medicine include a deep understanding of the physical structures and the energetic processes within the human body. Their understanding includes the ways qi and blood flow inside the channel system. The channel system includes *jing* and *mai.* Jing are the main channels. Mai are vessels—which are branches or collaterals of the main channels. The luo mai are the luo collaterals. The channels and collaterals are not only spaces where qi and blood flow, but are also areas where pathogens can lodge. As the body responds to pathogens, a set of unique signs and symptoms for each channel and collateral appears. The *Su Wen* and the *Ling Shu* present pathology created by imbalances in the luo mai, and list methods to treat them. Being able to identify a luo mai condition and direct a treatment at these collaterals is an important part of practicing acupuncture in a comprehensive and effective way.

The early Chinese medical practitioners discovered that the luo mai have two main functions:

1. The first function is to distribute qi and blood throughout the body.

2. The second function is to hold pathogenic factors.

The luo mai are outlets for pathogens in their own channels. Clinically, a main way to treat them is to prick to bleed to release pathogens. The luo mai can also be an outlet for other channels and their pathogens. In this situation, pathogens are moved from their channel system and area of the body to the superficial layer (the luo mai). The luo mai are then treated to remove the pathogen from the body. For example, if there was anger qi in the liver, a divergent channel treatment and/or a primary channel treatment can be applied to release the anger qi from the organ to the luo collaterals at the superficial level. The luo mai are then pricked to release the anger qi. As medical practitioners, we can work within the natural healing systems (which includes the acupuncture channels) of the body to safely and efficiently treat imbalances. This is the insight of the ancient practitioners of Chinese medicine. It is a gift from this ancient culture.

The main chapter on the luo mai is Chapter 10 of the *Ling Shu*, "The Main Channels." They are presented in detail in this chapter, including theory, diagnosis and clinical applications. The luo mai are also presented in a variety of chapters in the *Su Wen* and the *Ling Shu*. The *Ling Shu* is the definitive book on acupuncture. If there is a difference between the *Su Wen* and the *Ling Shu* regarding acupuncture, I refer to the *Ling Shu*. We will see how *Su Wen* passages are used to create theories and applications that differ from the *Ling Shu*. Important chapters in the *Su Wen* and the *Ling Shu* that provide essential information on the function and application of the luo collaterals will be introduced throughout this book.

TERMINOLOGY

The *Ling Shu* and the *Su Wen* present explanations of the luo mai. The *Ling Shu* is very clear in its presentation. There are chapters in the *Su Wen* that are the basis for new theories and clinical applications of the luo mai. Chapter 63 of the *Su Wen*, "Acupuncturing the Superficial Luo," is referenced to support new theories of the luo mai and the divergent channels. Chapter 63 is discussed in Chapter 9 of this book. The reader should critically evaluate the interpretations, theories and clinical applications that have been created based on this chapter.

Jing means "a channel."

Luo means "collaterals." These are branches off the main channels.

Luo means "connecting."

Mai means "a collateral."

Bie means "to divert or branch."

These meanings are an issue for our profession. Different translations (interpretations) can be used for different applications.

The luo mai are connecting collaterals. They are branches off the main channels (jing) and they help connect the small branches throughout the body. The luo mai are part of the integrated acupuncture channel system. The luo mai consist of the following layers:

1. *Bie luo.* These are the large luo mai. Bie luo are collaterals that divert or branch off the main channel. They begin at the luo point.
2. *Fu luo.* They are the floating or superficial luo; they are the blood vessels that are visible.
3. *Sun luo.* These are the grandchild or descendant luo. They are minute collaterals (small sub-branches) and are a couple of generations down from the bie luo.

LUO MAI FUNDAMENTALS

The *Ling Shu* describes the following fundamental qualities about the luo mai. There are a few *Su Wen* chapters referenced as well.

Luo mai paths

> Huang Di said, "The luo linking channels are unable to flow through the great joints. They must move by alternate routes to exit and enter; then they join again in the center of the skin. Their assemblies all can be seen from the outside."[3]

The luo mai are visible

> Lei Gong said, "How does one know the difference between the major channels and the luo linking channels?" Huang Di said. "The major channels cannot be seen. The 12 major channels lie hidden while traveling between the divisions of the flesh. They are deep and invisible, except for the Leg Major Yin, which passes through the upper part of the lateral anklebone and may be frequently seen because it has no place to hide."[4]
>
> "Those channels which float may be seen frequently and are the luo or linking channels."[5]
>
> "In all, there are 15 luo collaterals. When they suffer from a solid disease they become visible. When they suffer from a hollow disease, they sink."[6]
>
> "The channels that can be seen are all luo mai."[7]

The luo mai and temperatures

Cold

When the middle of the stomach is cold, the fish on the hand (the thenar eminence), the base of the thumb's linking collateral, will be mostly green-blue.

Hot

When the middle of the stomach is hot, the channels along the border of the fish (the thenar eminence) will be red.

Cold and hot

When the luo mai are red, black and green, it means both cold and hot qi.

Luo mai colors from the Ling Shu

> When the collaterals are blue or green, it indicates cold and also pain.
>
> When they are red, it indicates heat and fever.
>
> If there is an abrupt blackening of the luo collaterals, it is a sign of prolonged and chronic rheumatism.
>
> When they are red, black and green, it means both cold and hot qi.
>
> A green color and short indicates a sparseness of qi.
>
> A green-blue color located on the thenar eminence (fish on the hand) is cold in the middle of the stomach.
>
> A red color located on the border of the thenar eminence (fish on the hand) is heat in the middle of the stomach.

Luo mai colors from the Su Wen

In Chapter 57 of the *Su Wen*, colors of the luo mai are presented. This information is used to make a diagnosis of the luo mai.

The luo collaterals are more superficial than the main channels. The luo collaterals have colors that change: they can be green, red, yellow, white or black.

The colors of the main channels do not change, but the colors of the collaterals are variable.

The channels of the heart are red, the lung white, the liver green, the spleen yellow and the kidney black; each of the five organs has its individual correspondence to the five phases. *The color of the Yin collaterals always corresponds to their five phases.*

> The color of the Yang collaterals changes according to the seasons, for example, during the winter and autumn the cool temperature slows the flow of the blood and qi. It is common to see green, blue or

> black colors. The summer and spring are warmer and the heat causes a quicker flow of the blood and qi. It is common to see yellow and red colors in the luo collaterals. These seasonal color changes are normal. If all five colors show in the collaterals it indicates extreme cold or extreme heat; when this change is acute it is considered pathological.

The luo mai have no pulse

The main channels are measured with the pulse. The luo mai are not measured with the pulse. The following from the *Ling Shu* states that the main channels are measured with the pulse.

> If the main channels are hollow or solid, one must use the Inch Mouth (Renying Cukou pulse, located at Stomach 9 and Lung 9) to know.

Summary of the luo mai

- The luo mai are visible; their pathology can be identified by colors.
- The pulse does not measure the luo mai condition.
- The luo mai flow through the small articulations, not the big articulations.
- The luo mai are susceptible to heat and cold.

THE *SU WEN* AND THE LUO MAI

The *Su Wen* presents important aspects of the luo collaterals. Chapter 56 of the *Su Wen*, "Dermatomes of the Channels," describes the functions, signs, symptoms and pathology of the luo mai. Some of the main parts of this chapter are now presented.

Luo mai transferring pathogens

All diseases begin at the skin level. When a pathogen invades the skin, it forces the pores to open and it penetrates and lodges in the luo mai. If the pathogen is retained in the luo mai, it will transfer to the main channels. If the pathogen is not treated and removed from the main channels, it will then enter the fu (Yang) organs. One can determine where the disease is by observing the skin, the corresponding dermatomes and the luo mai. If one can see changes in the luo mai and does not treat them, the pathogen has the opportunity to flow to the internal organs and cause a major disease.

Before a pathogen enters the main channels it can be seen in the luo mai. The luo collaterals are considered Yang and they are located at the surface of the body. The main channels are considered Yin because they run relatively deep.

The chapter goes on to state that pathogens in each of the luo mai can be transmitted to the main channel or to the organs.

1. If the pathogen is excess, it will go to the main channels (if there is no proper treatment).
2. If the pathogen is Yang, it will be transmitted directly to the main channels.
3. If the pathogen is Yin, it will transfer to the channels and then the organs.

The chapter clearly expresses the view that the luo mai hold pathogens and describes how, if they are not treated, they can transfer deeper to the main channels (and the areas where they flow) and to the internal organs.

The *Su Wen* and *Ling Shu* chapters referenced describe essential aspects of the luo mai. It is vital to view the luo mai as a clinically important part of the acupuncture channel system. Understanding the role of each of the channel systems brings clarity to their functions and their clinical applications.

CHAPTER 2

THE LUO MAI PATHWAYS

THE CONNECTING COLLATERALS

The luo mai are a major part of the acupuncture channel system. The luo mai have specific pathways that are clearly described in the *Ling Shu.* There is a luo point for each of the 12 main channels, the Ren and Du channels, and the spleen has an additional luo mai and luo point. The *Su Wen* states that Stomach 18, Ru Gen, is also a luo point. It is commonly stated that there are 15 luo points. The *Nei Jing,* which includes both the *Su Wen* and *Ling Shu,* presents 16 connecting points.

The pathways of the luo mai are the areas where pathogens are located. The descriptions for the collaterals presented in this chapter are based on the *Ling Shu.* The pictures are modern illustrations of the descriptions. Evaluating the pathways and the signs and symptoms for these collaterals is the basis for a classical Chinese medicine diagnosis and treatment.

Chapter 17 of the *Ling Shu,* "The Limits of the Channels," says of the luo collaterals:

> The main channels make the foundation and the branches are horizontal and make the luo mai. These luo mai divide and make tiny vessels; when they are full with blood, quickly drain them.

The branches from the major channels are horizontal and they are the luo mai. These collaterals divide and make tiny vessels. A luo mai treatment influences this network.

THE LUO MAI PATHWAYS

The following luo mai descriptions are from Chapter 10 of the *Ling Shu*, "The Main Channels." The pictures offer an image of these written descriptions.[8] The areas in which the pathways flow can explain a large portion of the signs, symptoms and conditions of the luo mai. In parentheses are my comments for clarification.

The Arm Tai Yin luo mai (the lungs)

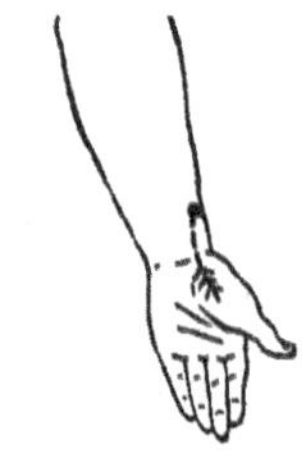

The luo mai branches off the Hand Tai Yin main channel at the point *Broken Sequence* (Lung 7). The luo mai starts above the wrist and runs parallel to the main Tai Yin channel (lungs). It penetrates into the palm and branches to the thenar eminence.

When there is an excess condition, it causes the wrist bone and palm to be hot. When there is a deficient condition, it results in yawning with the mouth open, and an increased frequency of urine.

Treat *Broken Sequence* (Lung 7). At this point a separate branch travels to the Bright Yang (large intestine).

The Arm Shao Yin channel (the heart)

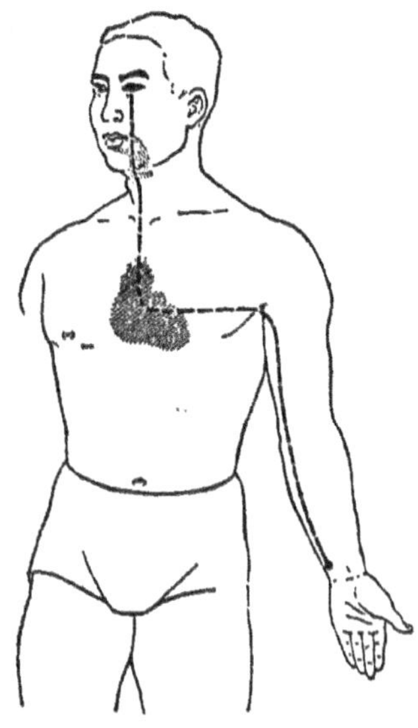

The Arm Minor Yin (heart) luo mai separates at the point called *Connecting Li* (Heart 5). It then travels up and follows the main channel to enter the middle of the heart, connects with the root of the tongue, and then makes connections to the eyes.

When there is an excess condition, there is a stick-like feeling in the chest (chest oppression). When there is a deficient condition, it can cause inability to speak.

Treat the *Connecting Li* (Heart 5) point. At this point a separate branch travels to the Major Yang (small intestine).

The Arm Jue Yin channel (the pericardium)

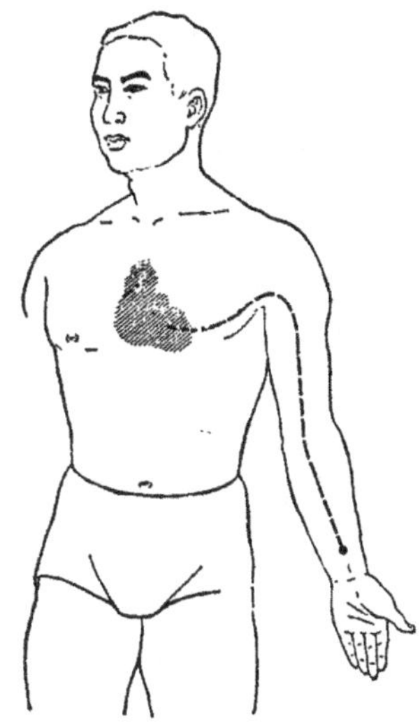

The luo mai separates at a point called *Inner Gate* (Pericardium 6). It flows upwards along the main channel to connect with the pericardium.

When there is an excess condition, there is pain in the heart. When there is a deficient condition, it causes rigidity of the head (cervical).

Treat the *Inner Gate* (Pericardium 6). At this point a separate branch travels to the Minor Shao Yang (san jiao).

The Arm Tai Yang channel (the small intestine)

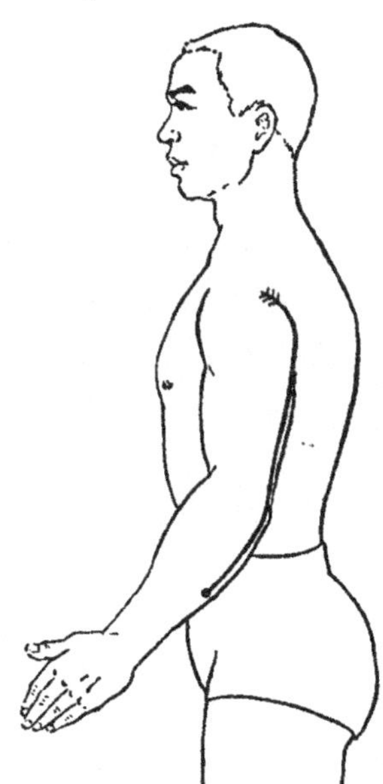

The luo mai of the Arm Major Yang (small intestine) separates at the point called *Branch to the Correct* (Small Intestine 7). A branch goes up to the elbow and connects with the shoulder bone point.

When there is an excess condition, there is a loosening of the joints and a wasting away of the elbow. When there is a deficient condition, there is growth of small swellings, including itching scabs.

Treat by using the *Branch to the Correct* (Small Intestine 7). At this point a branch flows to the Hand Shao Yin (heart).

The Arm Yang Ming channel (the large intestine)

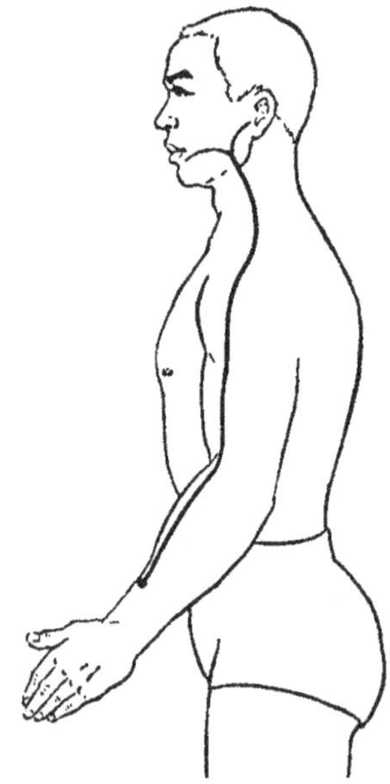

The luo mai of the Arm Bright Yang (large intestine) separates at a point called *Side Passage* (Large Intestine 6). A branch flows towards the Hand Tai Yin. Another branch follows the upper arm to the shoulder bone, then to the jaw and to the teeth. Another collateral enters the ear to join with the main channel.

When there is an excess condition, there is toothache and deafness. When there is a deficient condition, there is coldness of the teeth and obstruction of the diaphragm.

Treat *Side Passage* (Large Intestine 6).

The Arm Shao Yin channel (the san jiao)

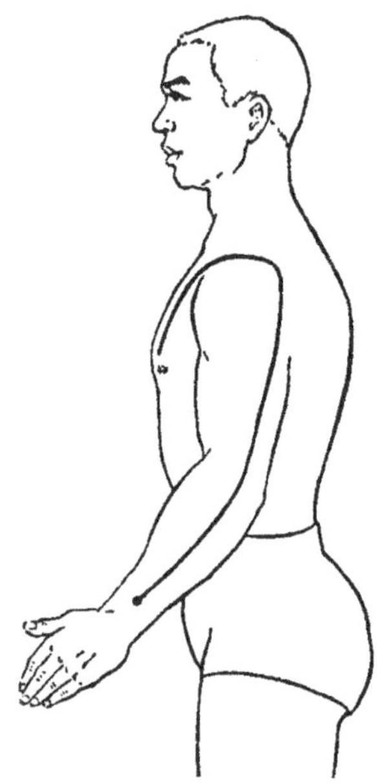

The luo mai of the Arm Minor Yang (san jiao) separates at *Outer Gate* (San Jiao 5). It flows up the arm and encircles the upper arm and shoulder to flow into the thorax.

When there is an excess condition, there is spasm of the elbow. When there is a deficient condition, there is the inability to crook.

Treat *Outer Gate* (San Jiao 5).

The Leg Tai Yang channel (the bladder)

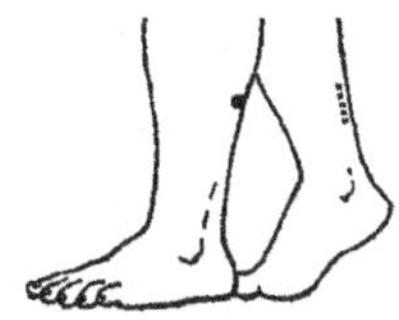

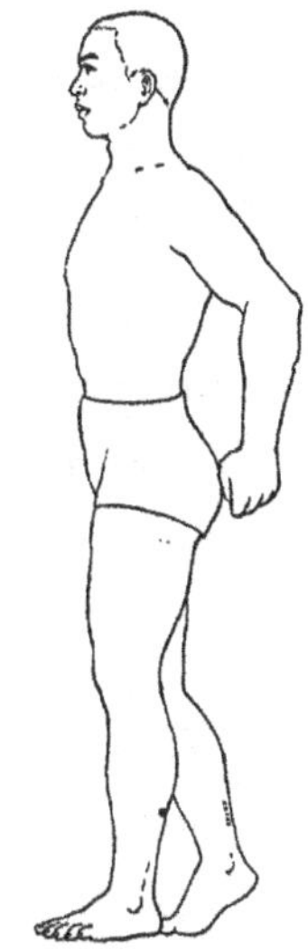

The luo mai of the Leg Major Yang (bladder) separates at a point called *Flying Yang* (Bladder 58). This luo mai travels to the Minor Yin (kidneys).

When there is an excess condition, there is a stuffed-up nose and pains in the head and back. When there is a deficient condition, there is a bloody nose.

Treat *Flying Yang* (Bladder 58).

The Leg Shao Yang channel (the gallbladder)

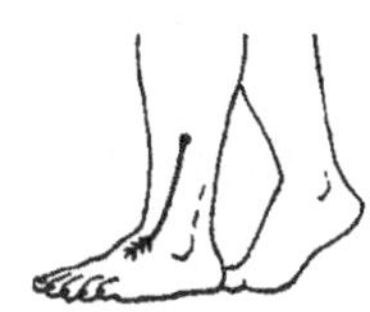

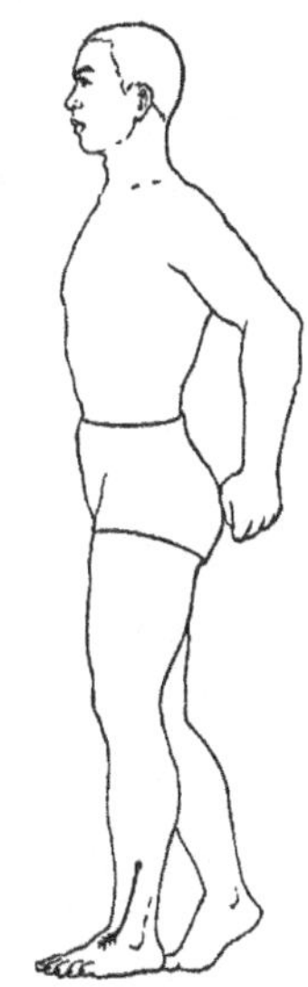

The luo mai of the Leg Minor Yang (gallbladder) separates at the point called *Bright Light* (Gallbladder 37). The luo mai separates and travels to the Shrinking Yin (liver). Another branch flows down toward the foot.

When there is an excess condition, there are cold feet. When there is a deficient condition, there is difficulty walking, paralysis and inability to rise from a sitting position.

Treat *Bright Light* (Gallbladder 37).

The Leg Yang Ming channel (the stomach)

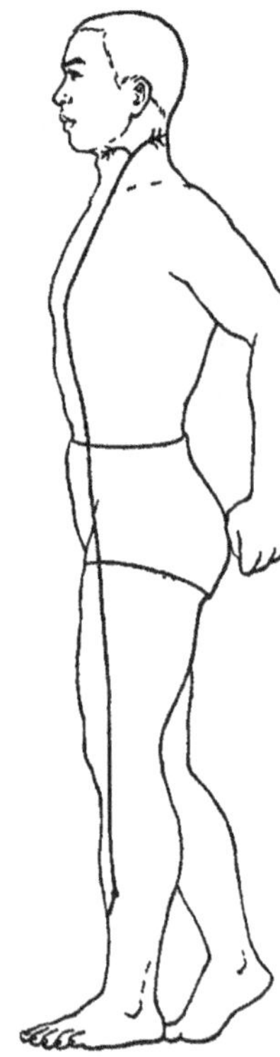

The luo mai of the Leg Bright Yang (stomach) separates at the point called *Abundant Bulge* (Stomach 40). The luo mai separates and flows to the Major Yin (spleen). Another branch flows along the main channel, then the lateral side of the leg bone; it then ascends to the neck and connects with the other channels in the area, and continues to the throat.

When the qi is rebellious counterflow, it results in numbness of the throat (sore throat) and a sudden loss of voice. When there is an excess condition, it causes madness. When there is a deficient condition, the foot is inflexible and the shin withers (paralysis of the lower limbs and atrophy of the legs).

Treat *Abundant Bulge* (Stomach 40).

The Leg Tai Yin channel (the spleen)

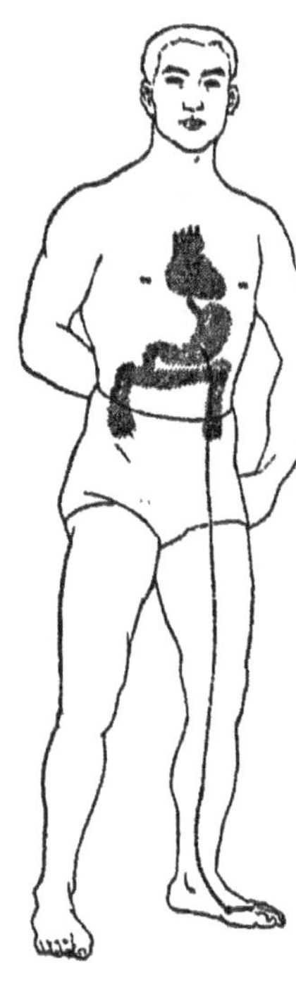

The luo mai of the Leg Major Yin (spleen) separates at the point called *Grandfather Grandson* (Spleen 4). A branch flows to the Leg Yang Ming channel. Another branch flows to the intestines and stomach.

When there is counterflow, there is vomiting and diarrhea. When there is an excess condition, it causes the middle of the Intestines to have sharp pains. When there is a deficient condition, there is drum-like swelling of the Intestines (abdominal swelling).

Treat at the *Grandfather Grandson* (Spleen 4).

The Leg Shao Yin channel (the kidney)

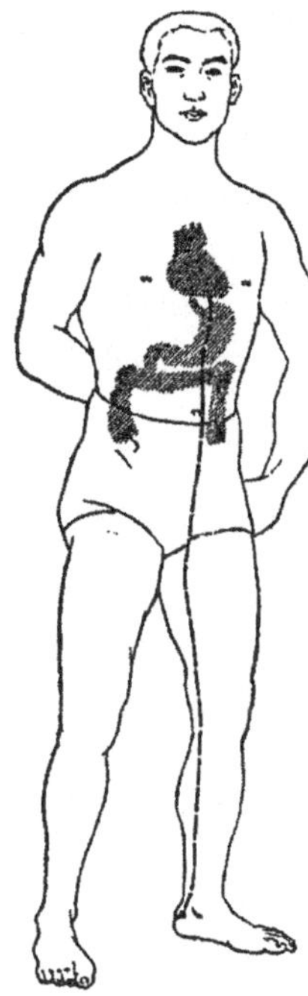

The luo mai of the Leg Minor Yin (kidney) separates at a point called the *Large Goblet* (Kidney 4). One branch travels to the Major Yang. Another branch flows with the main channel and ascends to the pericardium and then flows to the waist, the back and the spine.

When there is rebellious and counterflow qi, it causes annoyance and anxiety. When there is an excess condition, it causes blockage of urine. When there is a deficient condition, it causes pain in the loins and lumbago.

Treat *Large Goblet* (Kidney 4).

The Leg Jue Yin channel (the liver)

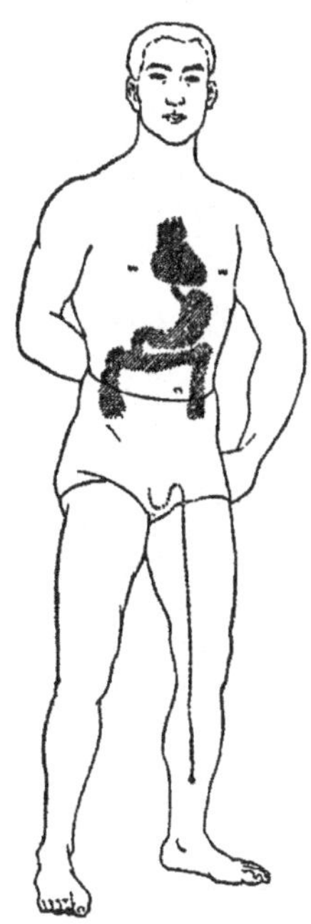

The luo mai of the Leg Shrinking Yin (liver) separates at the point called *Woodworm Canal* (Liver 5). A branch travels to the Leg Shao Yang. Another branch flows to the leg and ascends to the testicles and to the penis.

When the qi is rebellious, it creates swelling of the testicles and hernia. When there is an excess condition, there is an abnormal erection. When there is a deficient condition, there is itching.

Treat *Woodworm Canal* (Liver 5).

The Ren channel

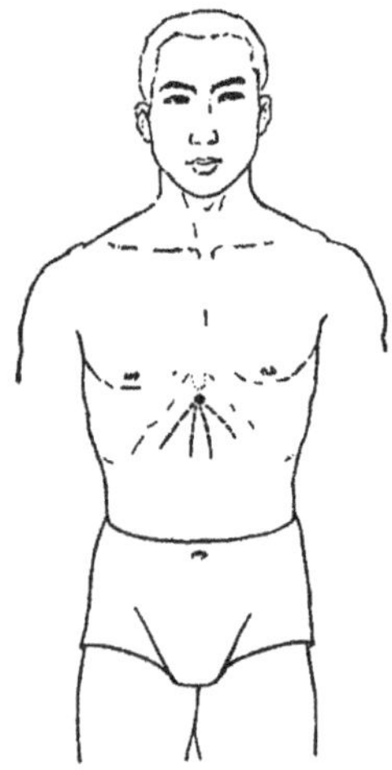

The luo mai of the Ren channel separates at *Dove Tail* (Ren 15). This luo mai begins below the xiphoid process and disperses to the abdomen.

When there is an excess condition, there is pain in the skin of the abdomen. When there is a deficient condition, there is itching along the luo mai area.

Treat *Dove Tail* (Ren 15).

The Du channel

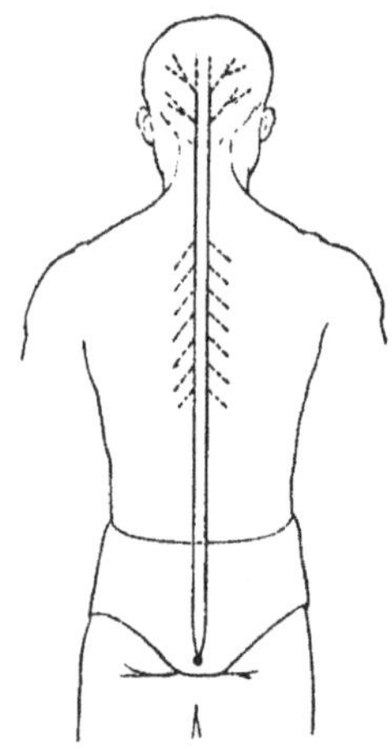

The luo mai of the Du channel separates at *Long and Strong* (Du 1). The collateral flows along both sides of the spine to the neck and spreads to the top of the head. The collateral then descends to the medial side of the scapula.

When there is an excess condition, there is rigidity of the spine. When there is a deficient condition, the head feels heavy.

Treat *Long and Strong* (Du 1).

The Great Luo channel (the spleen)

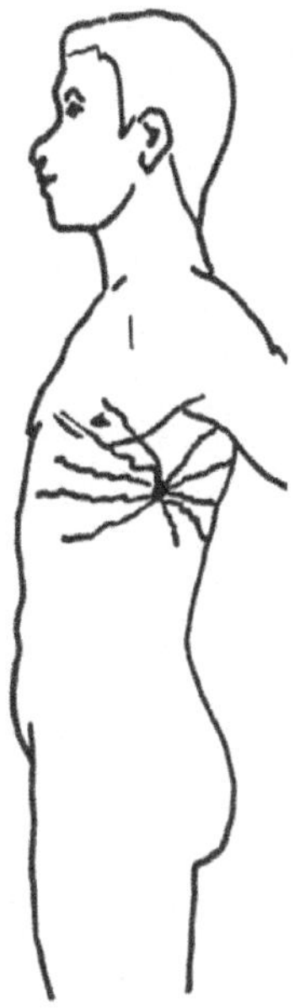

The great luo mai of the spleen starts at a point called *Great Wrapper* (Spleen 21). The luo main flows to the breast and the ribs.

When there is an excess condition, it causes pain in the whole body. When there is a deficient condition, it loosens a hundred joints. This luo mai controls the entire luo mai system and its blood.

Treat *Great Wrapper* (Spleen 21).

These 15 luo mai are the places where pathogens can be located and where the effects of pathogens can manifest. Pathogens create unique signs and symptoms that are presented in this chapter. These unique conditions correspond to individual luo mai and guide the practitioner to the specific luo mai to treat. This is a type of system of correspondences.

CHAPTER 3

THE LUO MAI FUNCTIONS AND CONDITIONS

The luo mai are primarily presented in Chapter 10 of the *Ling Shu*, "The Main Channels." These vessels are called the luo mai; the luo linking; the connecting vessels; or the luo collaterals. The chapter presents specific signs and symptoms in the luo mai, and states a treatment method, which is to treat the luo point. This knowledge is the classical clinical application of the luo mai found in Chapter 10 of the *Ling Shu*. The foundation information and functions of the luo mai are now presented.

- The luo mai are located in the superficial region of the body.
- The luo mai flow through the minor joints; they cannot flow through the main joints. (However, when a pathogen transfers to the main channels, it can flow into the main joints and wherever the main channels flow.)
- The luo mai can be visible. When pathogens are lodged in the luo mai they can be seen. Diagnosis includes visual examination of the luo mai. The main channels cannot be seen.
- The pulse does not detect the luo mai. The pulse does measure the main channels and the internal organs.
- Heat and cold are the main pathogens in the luo mai. Rheumatism occurs when pathogens in the luo mai are not treated effectively.
- The luo mai can have excess and deficiency conditions.

The *Su Wen* presents a few important aspects of the luo mai:

- The luo mai make up a protective channel system that can block and hold pathogens.
- Luo mai treatments release pathogens.
- Pathogens can be transferred from the luo mai to the main channels and the internal organs.

These functions are now presented in detail, with supporting theory from the *Su Wen* and the *Ling Shu*.

A PROTECTIVE SYSTEM

From the *Su Wen*, Chapter 56, "Dermatomes of the Channels."

> All disease begins at the skin level. When a pathogen invades the skin, it forces the pores to open and pathogens penetrate and lodge in the luo mai. If the pathogen remains it will transfer to the main channels. If the pathogen is not released it will then enter the fu organs.
>
> The function of the luo mai is to dispel pathogens and promote (allow) the normal flow of the ying and wei qi.
>
> Before a pathogen enters the main channels it can be seen in the luo mai. The luo mai are considered Yang and float to the surface; they can be seen. The main channels are considered Yin because they run relatively deep; they cannot be seen.[9]

This chapter goes on to say that if the pathogen is excess, it will be transmitted into the main channel. If it is a Yang pathogen, it will go to the channel. If it is a Yin pathogen, it will go first to the channel and then to the organ. This pattern occurs for all the channels.

From the *Su Wen*, Chapter 58, "Acupuncture Points."

> The collaterals that connect throughout the body act as connectors that can be utilized to release pathogens. They can also supply qi to

fight illness. There are 14 main collaterals, and there are numerous tiny collaterals crisscrossing the body, connecting the channels. If a pathogen enters the deep level of the bones, the collaterals are insufficient to treat this condition; the treatment must enter the five main channels of the five zang organs. The luo mai cannot treat this condition. (The luo mai are at the superficial level of the body.)[10]

LUO MAI PATHOGENS

The pathogenic factors of the luo mai are listed in the *Ling Shu*, Chapter 10, "The Main Channels," and in the *Su Wen*, Chapter 57, "The Channels and Collaterals." These pathogens and conditions are: cold, heat, rheumatism, qi stagnation and blood stagnation. Temperature, stagnation, deficiency, excess and the changes in the seasons can cause pathology in the luo mai. Heat and cold are the main pathogens in the luo mai. Pathology can show as colors. The changes of the seasons also cause reactions in the luo mai. The luo mai are especially susceptible to heat and movement generated by heat. The movement can transfer pathogens within the luo mai, and to other areas of the body. The luo mai are also susceptible to stagnation, which can lead to fever. The following are the main pathogens in the luo mai.

Heat

Heat and fever are a red color.

When the middle of the stomach is hot, the luo mai along the border of the fish (thenar eminence) will be red.

Cold

Cold and pain are a blue or green color.

When the middle of the stomach is cold, the fish on the hand (thenar eminence), the base of the thumb's luo mai, will be mostly green-blue.

Cold and heat

When there is both cold and hot qi, there is a red, black and green color.

Cold and heat are red, black and green.

Rheumatism

Rheumatism (bi syndrome) is a black color. It can be an abrupt blackening of the luo mai, and is a sign of prolonged and chronic rheumatism.

Luo mai and colors

- Blue is cold and pain.
- Green is cold and pain.
- Green-blue is cold in the stomach.
- Red is heat and fever.
- Sudden black is bi syndrome.
- Red, green and black is cold and heat.

Color, location and condition

Thenar eminence

- Blue at the thenar eminence is cold in the stomach.
- Red at the thenar eminence is heat in the stomach.
- Black at the thenar eminence is bi syndrome.
- Black, red and blue at the thenar eminence is cold and heat in the stomach.
- Blue is a short luo mai and is qi deficiency.

- Blackening is prolonged and chronic rheumatism.
- Green is a short collateral with sparse qi.

Table 3.1 Luo mai colors, locations and conditions

Color	Location	Condition
Green-blue	The fish on the hand (thenar eminence).	Cold in the middle of the stomach.
Red	Along the border of the fish (thenar eminence).	Heat in the middle of the stomach.
Blue	Short luo mai.	Qi deficiency.
Blackening	Abruptly showing in the luo mai.	Prolonged and chronic rheumatism.

Table 3.2 Luo mai colors and conditions

Color	Conditions
Blue or green	Cold, pain
Red	Heat, fever
Black (sudden)	Bi syndrome
Red, black and green	Cold and heat
Green	Channel is short, it is qi sparseness (qi deficiency)

Luo mai and the seasons

There are natural colors during the seasons and they are considered normal.

The Yin collaterals are the same color as their corresponding organs: the heart is red, the spleen is yellow, the lungs are white, the kidneys are black and the liver is green.

The Yang collaterals change color according to seasonal variations:

- During winter and autumn the cool temperature slows down the flow of the blood and qi. There can be green, blue and black colors.

- During the summer and spring it is warmer and heat causes a faster flow of the blood and qi. There can be a yellow and red color.

If the body displays all five colors in the collaterals, however, this indicates extreme cold or extreme heat. This acute change is considered pathological.

LUO MAI EXCESS AND DEFICIENCY

The luo mai can suffer from excess and deficiency conditions (shi and xu). The *Ling Shu* presents these two conditions for each of the luo mai. The guidance is that when the 15 luo mai are excess, they are visible, and when they are deficient, they sink. The practitioner should evaluate the luo mai to determine whether the condition is excess (solid) or deficient (hollow).

The following information for excess and deficiency is from the *Ling Shu*,[11] except when there is an asterisk, which designates the source is the *Jia Yi Jing*.

Excess and deficiency of the luo collaterals

THE ARM TAI YIN CHANNEL (LUNGS)

Excess: The wrist and palm are hot.

Deficiency: Yawning with the mouth open; frequent urination.

THE ARM MINOR YIN CHANNEL (HEART)

Excess: Pressure in the chest.

Deficiency: Inability to speak.

THE HAND JUE YIN CHANNEL (PERICARDIUM)

Excess: Pain in the heart.

Deficiency: Rigidity of the head. (Emotional upset.*)

The Arm Tai Yang channel (small intestine)

Excess: Loosening of the joints; wasting of the elbows.

Deficiency: Small swellings. These may be warts and scabs that itch.

The Arm Yang Ming channel (large intestine)

Excess: Toothache; deafness.

Deficiency: Coldness in the teeth; numbness in the diaphragm.

The Arm Shao Yang channel (san jiao)

Excess: Dysfunction of the elbow.

Deficiency: Dysfunction of the elbow.

The Leg Tai Yang channel (bladder)

Excess: Congested nasal passages; pain in the head and neck.

Deficiency: Bloody nose.

The Leg Shao Yang channel (gallbladder)

Excess: Deficiencies. Inversion.*

Deficiency: Paralysis, lameness; inability to rise from a sitting position.

The Leg Yang Ming channel (stomach)

When there is rebellious qi, there is a numb throat.

Excess: Madness. Manic. (Mania and withdrawal.*)

Deficiency: Inflexible foot. The shin withers. Flaccid muscles of the leg.

The Leg Tai Yin channel (spleen)

Excess: Sharp pains in the intestines; abdominal pain.

Deficiency: Swelling (drum-like) in the intestines; abdominal bloating.

The Leg Shao Yin channel (kidneys)

When there is rebellious and counterflow qi, there is depression and annoyance.

Excess: Constipation and blockage of urine.

Deficiency: Pain in the loins. (Low back pain.*)

The Leg Jue Yin channel (liver)

When there is rebellious and counterflow qi, there is swelling of the testicles and a hernia.

Excess: Abnormal erection.

Deficiency: Severe itching in the groin.

The Ren channel

Excess: Pain in the skin of the abdomen.

Deficiency: Itching in the abdomen.

The Du channel

Excess: Rigidity of the backbone; convulsions.

Deficiency: Heavy feeling in the head, and shaking at the top of the head.

THE GREAT LUO OF THE SPLEEN

Excess: Pain throughout the body.

Deficiency: All the joints are loose. (Slackness in the hundred joints.*)

The luo mai and the luo point control all the luo mai and their blood. Using this point can treat all the luo mai.

The luo mai make up a protective channel system. They hold or store pathogens and can be treated to release pathogens from the body. If the pathogens are not correctly treated, they may be transferred to the main channels, and possibly to the internal organs. They can also transform into bi syndrome. It is essential to treat pathogens before they transfer and cause a more serious condition.

Chapter 4

CLASSICAL CLINICAL APPLICATIONS

The *Ling Shu* is the earliest text on acupuncture. When the entire acupuncture channel system is used in clinical practice there is a clear understanding of the clinical applications of the luo mai. The *Ling Shu* presents clinical treatments for the luo collaterals. The main treatment is pricking, which is bloodletting. The objective of pricking is to remove pathogens from the body.

The treatment guidance in Chapter 10 of the *Ling Shu* is to treat the point of *separation of the luo mai*. The separation of the luo mai is the luo point on each channel. The name of the luo mai is the same as that of the luo point. For example, the Hand Tai Yin luo mai is Lie Que (Broken Sequence/Lung 7). When a diagnosis is made and a treatment plan is developed, the method is to prick the luo point on the diseased channel. There are three main methods of diagnosis:

1. diagnosis based on visual diagnosis
2. diagnosis based on the seasons
3. diagnosis based on excess and deficiency conditions.

TREATING THE LUO COLLATERALS

Chapter 10 of the *Ling Shu*, "The Main Channels," presents the following guidance:

> The way to treat the luo mai is bloodletting. Even if the pathogens cannot be seen, but there are symptoms, treat them to remove the pathogen by bloodletting. If the pathogen is not removed it can transform into rheumatism.[12]

Chapter 10 goes on to state:

> To use acupuncture for these cold and hot diseases, draw much blood from the luo collaterals. Treat once every other day. When this exhaustive bloodletting stops, then harmonize the hollow and the solid.[13]
>
> In extreme cases, to disperse results in depression. When depression is severe, it can result in fainting and in loss of speech; therefore, if there is depression, quickly seat the patient. When there is severe depression do not prick to bleed.[14]

The treatment for the luo mai is *prick to bleed.* There are three suggested places for treatment:

1. the point of separation (the luo point)
2. where there is a change in color in the luo mai
3. where the collaterals are twisted.

Note: "Twisted" can mean that a collateral is "full and firm, protuberant, dark red or purple in color."[15]

There is additional guidance:

> Therefore whenever one needles the network vessels, it is essential to hit the binding places. If it is severe, although there is as yet no blood binding (i.e. stasis) one must promptly treat the luo mai to drain (the pathogen) and remove the blood. If the pathogen is allowed to become lodged within the luo mai, this gives rise to bi.[16]

> Whenever needling cold and heat, one must treat the blood network vessels (by bleeding them), and this treatment must be performed once every other day until the blood is removed completely.[17]

> In all, there are 15 luo collaterals. When they suffer from a solid disease, they become visible. When they suffer from a hollow disease, they sink. Whether they are visible or invisible, one must investigate the complete circle, as well as top and bottom. People and channels both have their variations, so the luo linking channels have their differences and separations as well.[18]

> To use acupuncture for these cold and hot diseases, draw much blood from the luo collaterals. Treat once every other day. When this exhaustive bloodletting stops, then harmonize the hollow and the solid. When the channel is small and short, it means sparse qi. In extreme cases, to disperse results in depression. When depression is severe, it can result in fainting and in loss of speech; therefore, if there is depression, quickly seat the patient.[19]

Prick to bleed the point of separation (the luo point) is the main method for luo mai treatments. The treatment can be based on visual diagnosis, or on the excess and deficiency conditions of the luo mai. Chapter 10 of the *Ling Shu* presents the excess and deficiency conditions of the luo mai. Table 4.1 summarizes these conditions and lists the points of separation (luo points) that should be treated.

LUO MAI CONDITIONS

From the Ling Shu, Chapter 10, "The Main Channels"

In addition to making a diagnosis based on temperatures and colors, the excess and deficiency symptoms listed in Table 4.1 are the basis of diagnosis and treatment. The treatment is *prick to bleed the point of separation,* which is the luo point. Table 4.1 indicates the luo points used to treat the conditions set out in Chapter 3.

Table 4.1 The luo mai conditions and the luo points

Channel	Excess conditions	Conditions	The luo point to treat
Lung	Heat in the wrist and palm.	Yawning and frequent urination.	Lung 7
Heart	Fullness and pressure in the chest and diaphragm.	Loss of speech.	Heart 5
Pericardium	Heart pain.	Vexation in the heart.	Pericardium 6
Large intestine	Toothache, deafness.	Teeth sensitive to cold, bi conditions.	Large Intestine 6
Small intestine	Loosening of the joints and atony of the sinews in the elbow area.	Small swellings.	Small Intestine 7
San jiao	Spasms and cramps of the muscles around the elbow.	Atony of the elbows.	San Jiao 5
Stomach	Counterflow qi in the channel, throat bi and sudden loss of voice.	Atony of the feet and withering of the shins.	Stomach 40
Bladder	Nasal congestion with clear nasal discharge, headache, back pain.	Clear nasal discharge, bloody nose.	Bladder 58
Gallbladder	Inversion.	Weakness and atony of the lower limbs with inability to stand up from a sitting position.	Gallbladder 37

Spleen	Cholera, stabbing pain in the intestines.	Drum-like distension of the abdomen.	Spleen 4
Kidney	Vexation and oppression, constipation and urinary block.	Lower back pain.	Kidney 4
Liver	Swelling in the testicles, abnormal erection.	Sudden genital itching.	Liver 5
Ren	Pain in the skin of the abdomen.	Itching in the skin of the abdomen.	Ren 15
Du	Rigidity of the back.	Sensation of heaviness of the head, shaking the head.	Du 1
Great luo of the spleen	Aching and pain throughout the body.	Looseness of the hundred joints.	Spleen 21

The luo mai are an important part of the acupuncture channels system. The *Ling Shu* presents a framework to apply the luo mai in clinical practice. The luo mai hold pathogens. If the pathogens are not properly treated, they can transfer into the main channels, the internal organs and throughout the body. The following treatment locations for the luo mai follow the advice of the *Ling Shu*. The treatment for the luo mai is prick to bleed at the following locations:

1. the point of separation (the luo point)
2. where there is a change in color in the luo mai
3. where the collaterals are twisted.

Incorporating luo mai treatments into acupuncture practice can significantly increase clinical effectiveness. Targeting and treating the affected channel system is the central strategy in the classics of Chinese medicine. This includes the muscle channels, the luo collaterals, the main channels, the divergent channels and the eight extraordinary channels.

CHAPTER 5

THE SHEN

Lao Zi is considered the founder of philosophical Taoism. The *Tao Teh Ching* by Lao Zi is one of the most translated books in the world. The book describes the Way (Tao). It includes a profound description of what occurs when we do not follow the Way. The descriptions include a range of reactions to daily life, including emotional responses and psychological conditions. If the root of these responses and conditions is not changed, they can lead to a Shen disturbance. Lao Zi offers advice on how to find balance and live a natural and harmonious life, which is the path to living in harmony with the Way. Chinese medicine identifies exogenous and endogenous factors that influence the body, mind and spirit, and which can cause a Shen disturbance. The insights and life guidance from Lao Zi and specific Chinese medical practices for treating Shen disturbances are presented in this book. Integrating the two provides an effective framework for understanding and treating emotional imbalances and Shen disturbances.

Traditional Chinese medicine identifies conditions that can cause Shen disturbances. Certain conditions are organized by traditional Chinese medical patterns—for example, liver fire causing a liver hun and heart shen disturbance. The treatment plan is to clear liver fire and heart fire. A fantastic book that presents many of these patterns and syndromes is *Shen Disturbance: A Guideline for Psychiatry in Traditional Chinese Medicine*, by Joseph Changqing Yang (2005). I highly recommend this book for gaining an understanding of the traditional insight into Shen disturbances. Many people will get relief from psycho-emotional conditions and Shen disturbances by treating the patterns and the pathogens causing them.

The results can at times seem magical. This approach is part of the shift away from belief in supernatural intervention and performing exorcism.

THE *LING SHU* AND THE SHEN

"Shen" can be translated as "spirit." The ancient Chinese often described Shen in indirect ways. Instead of focusing on specific descriptions of Shen, they focused on how to experience Shen. Their focus is on Shen realization. They developed methods for people to practice (cultivation) that could guide them to Shen realization.

In Chapter 54 of the *Ling Shu*, "The Allotted Year of a Human's Life," Qi Bo is asked about the meaning of spirit (Shen). Qi Bo states:

> When one's blood and energy are complete and harmonized, when nourishing and protective qi are complete and penetrating, when the five viscera are complete and matured, the spirit qi is sheltered in the Heart and mind, and the animal spirit and human soul complete the organs, the person is complete.[20]

My interpretation of Qi Bo's answer is the following. Blood, nourishing qi and the animal spirit are Yin. Qi, wei qi and the human soul are Yang. The heart and mind are Yang, and the organs are Yin. When Yin and Yang are in harmony, vital substances, organs and emotions are in harmony, and the body and spirit are unified. This unification can lead to the following insight: when we are in balance and in harmony within ourselves and the world around us, our body and spirit naturally unify and we become a living expression of spirit (Shen realization), we are then complete. Shen realization is awareness of our most primary nature. This awareness is often called "aliveness." Taoists understand this aliveness as the most natural and fundamental aspect of a person. Qi gong, nei dan, acupuncture, herbal medicine and the *Tao Teh Ching* and the *I Ching* are ways to assist a person in their Shen realization.

Aliveness is described in a variety of ways. The most meaningful description for me is *present-awareness*. When we are aware, we are present with our aliveness. Thoughts, feelings and opinions appear and disappear; present-awareness always exists. Present-awareness is the Tao, and it is the Shen. Being fully aware (mindful of present-awareness) is Shen realization.

Qi Bo describes what makes a person complete. When we realize that we have present-awareness, we are complete. When we attach our identity to anything that is not present-awareness, we are incomplete. The severity of the attachment is a major cause of a Shen disturbance.

In the long history of China there have been numerous explanations of the cause of illness and Shen disturbances. The main causes according to early Chinese culture are presented below.

EARLY CHINESE CULTURE AND ILLNESS

The Shang dynasty is the first historic period of China. As in most ancient cultures, there was a belief in supernatural intervention. This belief is the basis of theurgic medicine. An example of theurgic medicine in China is the "curse of the ancestors," which is the first main explanation of illness in the Shang dynasty. This explanation includes the belief that there is a relationship between the living and the dead, and that if a living person attacked or harmed another living person, the harmed person's ancestors would harm the attacker, causing illness. We could evaluate this theory as a cultural explanation to guide people's behavior. The goal is to get people to act in ways that create harmony among the living. With harmony on earth, there would be harmony with the ancestors.

In the Zhou dynasty, the second historic period, a new explanation of illness was introduced. During the Warring States period (403–221 BC) of the Zhou dynasty, civil war occurred in China. This period was the most violent in its history. The Chin tribe and its leader Ying Zheng were at the center of the warring period. His goal was to conquer all the tribes in the country and unify China under his sole control. Within this unification he would become the first emperor of China. The Warring States period included violent chaos. In the Chinese view, the violent chaos on earth caused violent chaos in the heavens (the ancestors). The chaos broke the direct bond between the living and the ancestors. This broken bond led to demons or ghosts, which did not follow any ancestor relationship. The ghosts or demons would attack anybody. In the same way that the warring armies attacked anybody in their pursuit of defeating all on their way to total domination, so demons or ghosts could attack anybody. Medicine to treat demons became part of the culture, and exorcism became a main treatment method. Currently, the oldest known Chinese medical book is the Mawangdui medical texts, which are from the Warring States period of the Zhou dynasty. Curse of the ancestors and attack by demons were a main explanation of illness and Shen disturbance at that time.

From the Warring States period to the Han dynasty, there was a transformation in Chinese medicine. The Han dynasty classics, the *Su Wen* and the *Ling Shu*, developed from the Mawangdui medical texts. Practitioners added new and more detailed information about nature, the human body and the channels. Most importantly, they added acupuncture points to the Mawangdui texts. One area in which the *Su Wen* and the *Ling Shu* shifted away from the Mawangdui texts was the belief in curse of the ancestors and demons as a cause of illness. The *Su Wen* and the *Ling Shu* medical texts include a sophisticated analysis of the causes of illness based on genetics (jing), external pathogenic factors, internal pathogens and lifestyle. There is a magnificent presentation of the cycles and patterns of nature in the classics (see Chapters 66–71 of the *Su Wen*). The books present cycles of days, months and years that create pathogens not commonly known to the average person or medical practitioner (atmospheric influences). It is possible to view genetic/jing conditions as a type of curse of the ancestors. If demons are viewed as illnesses or conditions that arise from an unknown cause, the pathogens created by invisible (atmospheric influences) cycles of time can be viewed as a variation of the influence of demons or ghosts. These cycles of nature are a more modern way of explaining these unknown influences.

In early Chinese philosophy books, as well as the classic medical texts the *Su Wen* and the *Ling Shu*, Shen is often explained in nebulous ways. The books generally explain the actions of life that cause an imbalance of Shen, and ways to restore balance and harmony. In the *Su Wen* and the *Ling Shu* there are detailed diagnoses based on Chinese medical principles. When a person has a Shen disturbance, the condition/s are usually explained using Chinese medical patterns and syndromes—for example, liver fire, or phlegm misting the heart. A treatment is made based on Chinese medical principles. Treatment can include herbs, acupuncture, dao yin (qi gong), nutrition and lifestyle guidance. The contributors to the *Nei Jing* do not deny other causes of Shen disturbance; they present a significant, deep and profound model of evaluation that allows the practitioner to apply healing methods within the *Nei Jing* medical system that may help a certain percentage of people. For other causes of Shen imbalances, therapy, spiritual guidance and western medicine can be an important part of the treatment and healing process.

Chinese and Taoist healers have several ways of viewing Shen. A common way is viewing the overall condition of a person; for example, their Shen is strong, or the Shen is disturbed. The Shen can also be viewed in two aspects, i.e. Yin–Yang, and the Hun and Po. The Hun is the Yang and ethereal aspect of a person, and the Po is the Yin and corporeal aspect. Another way to view Shen is the *five shen*. The five shen is an important medical framework for diagnosis and treatment. The five shen will be presented in detail in this book.

THE WAY

The ancient Chinese people studied nature deeply. They perceived the cycles of human development and nature's endless flows and cycles. They observed the visible world. They were also able to perceive the invisible forces within the visible world, and they mapped out the invisible energetic forces of nature. They understood that the invisible and the visible are one inseparable whole. These ancient people viewed the creator and creation as one. The creative force of the universe is within all of life. The Chinese named the entire process, function and structure of the world the *Tao*. The Tao includes the invisible forces and visible forms of the world. The cycles and flows of the visible world contain a force, which they called qi. Tao includes qi. All of life is the Tao, and the Tao is within all of life. When a person is aware of this reality they are aware of the Tao within themselves. The Tao within each person includes the Shen. A definition of a Shen imbalance or disturbance includes no awareness of the Tao (Shen). This lack of awareness can arise from a deep polarity within a person and is a main cause of illness.

The *Tao Teh Ching* is the foundation for all traditions of Tao. The following is from Chapter 25 of the *Tao Teh Ching*.

Before Heaven and Earth are born,
there is something formless and complete in itself.
Impalpable and everlasting, silent and undisturbed,
standing alone and unchanging,
It exercises itself gently,
and generates itself inexhaustibly in all dimensions.
It may be regarded as the Mother of all things.
Far beyond humans' relative conception,
it cannot be referred to by a specific name.
Yet it may be identified as the Tao,
the subtle truth of the universe.
Expressing its integral nature,
Tao remains intangible, yielding, and uncontrollable: the ultimate expression of the cosmos.
As an expression of its unceasing creativeness,
it first manifests as the spaciousness of the sky.
As an expression of its receptiveness,
it manifests second as the great massiveness of galaxies, stars, and planets.
As a further expression of its harmonious reintegration,
it manifests third as human life.
Thus, in the natural flow of energy transformation,
human life becomes of the four great expressions of the path of subtle universal integration.
Humankind confirms itself to Earth.
Earth confirms itself to the sky.
The sky confiorms itself to the Subtle Origin.
The Subtle Origin confirms to its own nature.[21]

This chapter of the *Tao Teh Ching* includes the insight that the creator of the universe is within its creation. When someone confirms and aligns oneself with earth (the Tao), they realize that they are part of creation and inseparable from the Tao. This process of confirming, aligning and attuning to Shen is called "Shen realization." The ancient Chinese have developed numerous ways to assist in Shen realization. The ways include meditation, nei dan (inner alchemy), prayer, qi gong, acupuncture, herbal medicine and reading classics (*I Ching*, *Tao Teh Ching*, etc.). Some of the Shen realization methods are simple and some are very complex. A variety of ways to assist a person in Shen realization is presented in the following chapters.

THE SHEN

All of humanity share living on planet Earth; it can be called *aliveness*. Every person can have *awareness* of this aliveness. This awareness is often described as mystical, magical and transcendental. In reality, it is the most natural and normal part of life. This aliveness is Shen. It is also called the Original Shen (Original Spirit). Chinese spiritual and medical traditions have numerous ways to assist a person in attuning to this aliveness. Stress, trauma and conditioning (life experiences) that occur in our life can shift our consciousness away from awareness of aliveness.

A DIAMOND IN THE ROUGH

A diamond in the rough is an image that illustrates how the process of Shen realization (self-realization) can occur. Each person has a diamond. The diamond is the Shen. The rough includes the stresses, conditioning, imprints, patterns, emotions and unfavorable influences that exist in our life. We all have a diamond shining within, and we all have rough. The amount and types of rough vary among people. Acupuncture can assist in releasing, clearing and removing the rough, thereby allowing insight and alignment with the diamond. This process can be life-changing, and can provide additional inspiration and motivation for further changes. It can inspire a person to live in a way that allows synchronization with Shen (becoming aware of it) and becoming a living expression of Shen.

JING–SHEN

The Chinese understood that life experiences could shift awareness away from Shen. Sometimes there are minor shifts, and sometimes there are major shifts. These people expressed their understanding of the integration of the relationship of Shen and life experiences with the term *Jing–Shen*. Jing is the physical body and the experiences we have processed and retained in our body–mind. It is these experiences and our response to them that can either maintain our Shen awareness, or cause a shift away from it. Jing–Shen contains an accumulation of experiences and their influences on our life. In spiritual cultivation, a goal is to clear away or understand the experiences in our life that cause a Shen disturbance. This process can allow Shen realization.

Jing is the physical aspect of a person, and Shen is the spiritual part. These two aspects of a person are one inseparable whole. Each influences the other. Our experiences of life are stored in Jing, and Jing influences the Shen. Jing influences how we perceive, respond and interact with all aspects of our life. This symbiotic relationship reflects the way we experience life based on the environment while in the womb, our early childhood experiences, and conditioning from our family and society. The body processes these experiences, and if all is well they are filtered in a way that allows us to grow, mature and develop in a favorable way. Often our experiences are difficult and can be traumatic. Jing holds the experiences, which can then influence our ability to connect and align with Shen. As medical practitioners, we can apply the methods of Chinese medicine to assist a person in restoring balance and harmony in their life by reducing/releasing the held, unfavorable experiences. This releasing can allow awareness and natural expression of the Shen.

In the following chapters qi gong, luo collateral treatments and other acupuncture channel treatments are presented to assist in releasing stagnations, trauma and conditioning that may have entered Jing–Shen. The methods presented are practical approaches to assist a person in achieving physical health, psycho-emotional balance and spiritual realization.

CHAPTER 6

THE FIVE SHEN

Chinese culture is one of the most diverse in the world. Chinese traditions include indigenous culture, shamanism, Taoism, Confucianism, Buddhism and combinations of all of them. Each tradition has a unique insight about life. And each tradition has an understanding of spirit. The Chinese word for spirit is "Shen." From a macro viewpoint each person has one Shen. We can view the totality of a person in terms of one Shen. This would include the general psycho-emotional and spiritual condition of a person. For example, we might say that person has a vibrant Shen. We might also say they have a Shen disharmony. The term encompasses the collective condition of a person. The Chinese also view the Shen as multi-dimensional. The multi-dimensional view of a person is the *five shen.*

Chinese medicine offers a model that can view each person both as a whole and in component parts, which allows diagnosis of these two aspects of a person. A person can be viewed in terms of their physical parts to target their physical condition. For example, a medical practitioner can evaluate a person's muscles, bones, arteries, veins, glands and the internal organs to identify which of these may be diseased. The Shen can also be evaluated according to its parts. Viewing the Shen both as the collective condition of a person and in its parts (its multi-dimensional form) is part of Chinese spiritual and medical traditions. The contributors to the *Ling Shu* and the *Su Wen* left a road map of these traditions; both are valuable in clinical practice.

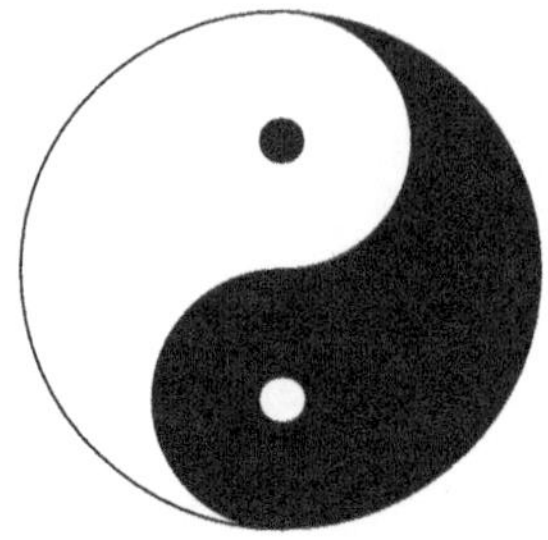

Figure 6.1 The Tai Chi symbol

Tai Chi is a model to explain how the universe (Tao) functions. Tai Chi contains three forces: Yang, Yuan and Yin. In Figure 6.1 the white color is Yang, the black color is Yin and the curved line down the middle is Yuan. Yuan is the original force; in this case it is the original energy. This original energy can be understood in terms of expansion into Yin and Yang. The three forces are really one integrated force. These three forces interact to create an infinite number of patterns that comprise the universe. This is the macrocosmic view of Tai Chi. The microcosmic view is that the Tao divides the whole into three component parts known as the *three treasures*. These treasures are Jing, Qi and Shen. Like the three forces in the Tai Chi symbol, the three treasures are inseparable. Each treasure can be viewed, evaluated and treated as an individual treasure. Each treasure can also be viewed as one part of an interrelated process where each one influences the others.

The human body contains the Yin–Yang organ pairs (the pericardium and the san jiao are not grouped as organs). Likewise, the Shen can be understood in terms of its relationship to each of these organ pairs. The relationship of the Shen to the organs is represented as the five shen. Chinese medicine includes a unique insight that the five Yin organs house the five shen. This insight is an example of the interrelationship between the body and mind.

Chinese medicine distinguishes the functions and imbalances of the Shen from the five shen. A way to communicate this difference is to capitalize the S in "Shen" when referring to the collective aspect of the spirit. The five shen will be lower case: for example, the shen, the yi, the po, the zhi and the hun of the heart, spleen, lungs, kidneys and the liver. The five shen are five aspects of the one Shen.

The five Yin organs provide vital substances to maintain life. Each of the five organs also has a function and role in health and vitality. Most interestingly, the ancient healers perceived the resonance between the five Yin organs and the psycho-emotional condition. These healers created the five shen Chinese medical model to explain this relationship.

The following passage from Chapter 5 of the *Su Wen* describes a relationship between nature, the internal organs and the five shen.

> Nature contains the four seasons and the five phases of wood, fire, earth, metal, and water. The five phases interact, change, and transform to create cold, summer heat, damp, dryness, and wind. The weather affects everything in the natural world and is the foundation for the cycle of life: birth, growth, maturation, and death. In the human body there are the five yin (zang) internal organs of the Heart, Spleen, Lungs, Kidneys, and the Liver. The organs provide the structure and the qi to form and allow the manifestation of the five spirits, which then gives rise to the five natural virtues and emotions.[22]

This *Ling Shu* passage explains the materialization of the five shen in the body. The description expresses the relationship between the cosmos and humanity: the macrocosm and microcosm. Chapter 8 of the *Ling Shu* presents the five shen and their relationships to the five Yin organs. The psychological, emotional and mental qualities of each organ are presented. The condition of the organs can influence the five shen and their related areas of life; conversely, the condition of the five shen (psycho-emotional) can influence the organs. For example, fear can manifest if someone has a chronic kidney deficiency.

The *Ling Shu* reference quoted above describes the interrelationship between the Yin organs and the five shen. The Yin organs create the structure for the five shen to manifest in life, which includes their corresponding virtues. The organs provide the physical structure for the five shen to exist in the body. This is a foundation relationship for the body/mind/spirit relationship and holistic medicine.

The five shen medical model provides a clinically effective framework to treat psycho-emotional conditions. It provides a system that enables the practitioner to match specific psycho-emotional conditions to their corresponding channels, points, vital substances and energy centers in the body. These relationships allow the practitioner to customize a treatment for each patient.

There are two main ways to diagnose a Shen condition. The first is by assessing the overall condition of a person; and the second is by assessing the five shen. One or more of the five shen can be imbalanced. A goal in treatment is to restore each of the five shen, creating a balanced Shen.

The five shen model enables the practitioner to make a targeted treatment, which in my experience is more effective than applying only a general Shen treatment. Treating any of the five shen with their corresponding luo point is a direct way to influence that organ/shen correspondence. This method is especially effective when the psycho-emotional condition is *active* and disturbing. It is also an effective way to assist in releasing repressed emotions and experiences. In that situation, the luo points can be used with other channel systems to treat the psycho-emotional condition.

The *Ling Shu* and the *Su Wen* include detailed information about the five shen. The following section explains the foundation for a "five shen" diagnosis and treatment plan.

THE FIVE SHEN

Chapter 5 of the *Su Wen*, "The Manifestation of Yin and Yang from the Macrocosm to the Microcosm," presents the five shen. The five shen are a model for understanding patterns of disharmony. The ancients understood that the Yin organs house the five shen; Yang (shen) must have Yin (organs) to contain it. The conditions of the five shen can influence the Yin organs, and the conditions of the Yin organs can influence the five shen.

A strategy for treatment is matching emotion(s) to their corresponding shen and organ. In the metaphor of the diamond in the rough, imbalances of these emotions are *the rough*. Acupuncture (and pricking to bleed) can assist in clearing the roughness, revealing the shining light of the diamond (i.e. the Shen). Awareness of your Shen can inspire, motivate and provide the incentive for change and transformation.

Five shen resonances

Five shen resonances (correspondences) tell us much about the nature of the five shen. The main resonances are from the *Ling Shu*, Chapter 8, "Roots and Spirit," and the *Su Wen*, Chapter 5, "The Manifestation of Yin and Yang from the Macrocosm to the Microcosm."

The twelve organs

- The heart is the sovereign of all organs and represents the consciousness of one's spirit. It is responsible for intelligence, wisdom and spiritual transformation.
- The lung is the advisor. It helps the heart in regulating the qi.
- The liver is like the general. It is intelligent and courageous.
- The gallbladder is like a judge. It has the power of discrimination.
- The pericardium is like the court jester. He makes the emperor laugh, bringing joy.
- The stomach and spleen are like warehouses; they store food and essences. They digest, transform and transport food and nutrients.
- The large intestine transports turbidity (waste products).
- The small intestine receives the food that has been digested by the spleen and stomach; it further extracts, absorbs and transports the food's essences from the extraction process throughout the body. It separates the pure from the turbid.
- The kidneys store vitality. This mobilizes the four extremities. The kidneys also benefit the memory, willpower and coordination.
- The san jiao promotes the transformation and transportation of fluids throughout the body.
- The bladder is where water converges and is eliminated.

The five storehouses

- The liver is the storehouse of blood and it is the shelter of the human soul (hun spirit).
- The spleen is the storehouse of nourishment and it is the shelter of thought (yi spirit).
- The heart is the storehouse for the channels and it is the shelter of the spirit (shen spirit).
- The lung is the storehouse of qi and it is the shelter of the animal spirit (po spirit).
- The kidneys are the storehouse of the seminal essence and they are the shelter of the will (zhi spirit).

The five shen and their inherent qualities

- The spirit of the heart is called the shen and it rules mental and creative functions.
- The spirit of the liver is called the hun and it rules the nervous system and gives rise to extrasensory awareness.
- The spirit of the spleen is known as the yi and it rules logic and rational thought.
- The spirit of the lungs is called the po and it rules the animalistic instincts, and physical strength and endurance.
- The spirit of the kidneys is called the zhi and it rules the will, drive, ambition and the survival instinct.

The five shen and emotions

- Anger can injure the liver; but sadness can relieve anger. Metal controls wood. The po controls the hun.

- Too much joy can cause a depletion of the heart qi. This can be counterbalanced by fear. Water controls fire. The zhi controls the shen.
- Excessive worry will deplete spleen qi; but anger can restrain this worry. Wood controls earth. The hun controls the yi.
- Extreme grief can injure the lungs; but it may be countered by the emotion of happiness. Fire controls metal. The shen controls the po.
- Fear and fright will damage the kidneys. They can be defeated with understanding, logic and rational thinking. Earth controls water. The yi controls the zhi.

In applying the last set of five-phases relationships, the controlling cycle is identified to treat an imbalance. In my experience, when the controlling cycle is in balance, the controlling phase shapes the controlled phase. For example, the zhi (water) shapes the shen (fire). It shapes it by sending its balanced energy and its virtues to the heart (shen), bringing it into balance. This shaping occurs for all the five shen.

Some practitioners apply this controlling (shaping) theory to the five transporting points to treat emotional conditions. The Han dynasty classic medical text, the *Nan Ching* (*The Classic of Difficulties*), introduces the five phases points (the five element points); they are not presented in the *Su Wen* or the *Ling Shu*. In this method, the imbalanced organ is identified and its controlling phase is needled. For example, if a person has anger and is irritable, the metal point on the liver channel is treated: Liver 4, Middle Seal, the metal point on the liver channel, is treated to relieve anger. Anger can injure the liver, but sadness can relieve anger. Sadness is the emotion of the lungs, which is metal. Metal can relieve anger, in this theory. This principle can be applied to all the channels.

The knowledge of each of the five shen has important clinical value. When there is an imbalance of the emotions, the practitioner can match the emotion to its corresponding organ and shen. These connections are the foundation for an organ and a five shen diagnosis and treatment plan.

The following insight from the *Ling Shu*, Chapter 8, "Roots and Spirit," is important in clinical practice:

> When the Heart and mind is frightened and full of distressed thoughts and anxiety, it can result in injury to the spirit. This can result in fear and loss of self.[23]

This quote can be interpreted in the following way: with stress and emotional turmoil we can lose awareness and connection to self (spirit). Acupuncture can assist in clearing or releasing the emotional attachment to the stress and turmoil. The release can assist in helping a person reconnect with their spirit. This process is sometimes called self-realization.

The five shen are an example of the ancient healers' and spiritual practitioners' awareness of the unity of the body, mind and spirit. Five shen correspondences of the internal organs are presented in the *Su Wen*, Chapter 5, "The Manifestation of Yin and Yang from the Macrocosm to the Microcosm," and Chapter 8, "The Sacred Teachings." This information is essential in making a diagnosis and developing a treatment plan. The key is to identify imbalances and the conditions that cause them. Often the emotional, psychological and spiritual condition reveals areas of life that a person needs to understand in order to grow. It is common for a person to act in a way that causes the imbalances to be expressed in their life; this expression may be necessary to raise awareness of the condition. The awareness provides an opportunity to recognize the situation and begin a path of change and transformation. The practice of Chinese medicine, including acupuncture, herbs and qi gong, can assist in this path of change, transformation and self-realization.

The five shen and their paired organs

The five shen model includes the five Yin–Yang paired organs. For example, when the heart shen is mentioned, it refers to the heart and the small intestine. Below we look at each.

THE HEART (SHEN)

The heart houses the heart shen and the Shen. The heart shen corresponds to the physical and psycho-emotional conditions of the heart organ. (The Shen is also called the original shen—the yuan shen, "the diamond.")

Methods that connect a person to their heart shen can provide the opportunity to realize knowledge, inspiration, wisdom and guidance regarding their spirit. Attuning to the heart shen can bring direct experience of spirit and the inseparable nature of the universe. This unity exists for all people. In Chinese culture, living from this awareness is called Wu Wei, which can be translated as "nothing extra." It is sometimes translated as "no-thing." "Nothing extra" means that we add no extra opinions, thoughts, beliefs and preconceived ideas to our direct experience of our essential nature (spirit). To live in the Tao is to live from our spirit, and the way to do this is by living in Wu Wei.

From an acupuncture pathway viewpoint, the Chong and kidney pathways connect the kidneys and the heart. The kidneys house Jing and the heart houses the Shen; this unity is called Jing–Shen. The channel flow reveals that there is a circuit of channels that form a pathway to the heart shen. This pathway to the heart shen can be accessed at any time. As healthcare practitioners, we can assist in helping our patients realize their Shen (self-realization) by treating this channel pathway.

The Shen includes the small intestine and heart's innate quality of living a natural life. The experiences of this fire system can include experiencing the unity of life, which can be a transcendental experience. With time this awareness of the unity of life becomes normal and part of everyday life. Stagnation, blockages and repression of this aspect of life can manifest in intense outward expressions, which can be physical or emotional. For example, yelling, screaming, punching or emotional outbursts can occur at any time, reflecting the volatile and explosive nature of fire.

The heart opens to the tongue. Shen imbalances can manifest in the way one speaks. The imbalance can include too much talking or the inability to express oneself clearly. A disconnect from spirit can occur, which can lead to a loss of passion for life. This type of separation can lead to bitterness (the taste and quality of the heart).

Connecting to our heart shen is a primary experience in many spiritual traditions. As practitioners of the healing arts, assisting others in making this connection or realization is one of the most powerful and life-changing experiences for both the practitioner and the patient.

The kidneys (zhi)

The kidneys house the zhi shen, which corresponds to jing and genetics. Ancestral medicine is one of the oldest sources of medicine in China. It originates in the Shang dynasty. During this time the Chinese viewed the living and the deceased as existing simultaneously; most importantly, they influence each other. (A modern interpretation of this influence is genetics.) It can also include the culture, religion and beliefs of family, caretakers and those with an influence during early life. Transcending any unfavorable effects of those influences is essential to living a fulfilling life. If they are not transcended, they can lead to increased stagnation and rigidity. They can freeze a person.

Zhi relates to willpower. It includes the will and power to follow one's destiny. The kidneys loathe cold, which can freeze water and change its essential nature of adaptability and flexibility. The kidney channel flows up the front of the body to the chest through the heart area. This pathway is one example of zhi seeking shen. It is a built-in energetic system in each person. If there is a freezing or rigidity due to conditioning, we may not be able to have a full life. The freezing can change the flowing and adaptive nature of each person, blocking awareness of his or her Shen.

A goal in life should be to allow expression of the issues related to the freezing of the zhi. Expression allows for freeing up stagnations and blockages. For example, if a person wanted to be an artist but did not pursue it, a part of them is suppressed or repressed. The suppression can lead to a deep polarity. If a person pursues artistic activities, it allows important qualities of the person to be experienced, allowing a free flow of energy. The expression is a type of letting go. Letting go can create a space (awareness) which can be a place of change and transformation. Chapter 11 of the *Tao Teh Ching* expresses this subtle truth:

> Thirty spokes together make a wheel for a cart. It is the empty space in the center of the wheel which enables it to be used.
>
> Mold clay in a vessel. It is the emptiness within that creates the usefulness of the vessel.
>
> Cut out doors and windows in a house. It is the empty space inside that creates the usefulness of the house.

> Thus, what we have may be something substantial,
>
> But its usefulness lies in the unoccupied, empty space.
>
> The substance of your body is enlivened by maintaining the part of you that is unoccupied.[24]

The empty space in us is created when we let go of stagnations and blockages, allowing us to focus (mindfulness) on our present-awareness. This awareness is the empty space described in Chapter 11 of the *Tao Teh Ching*. The empty space is a way of describing the most essential part of every person. The Chinese call this empty space Shen. Awareness of this empty space is Shen realization.

The zhi and jing represent unlimited possibilities. In Chinese philosophy, we call this "chaos" or Wu Ji, which is a state or qi field where anything is possible. And it is awareness or an openness that allows anything to manifest. No limits are placed on it. This space is inside each person. When we live from this space there is no freezing or rigidity placed on the kidneys, jing and the zhi (the organ, substance and shen). If our ancestral influences (genes) or our family postnatal influences freeze or block our ability to be open to all possibilities, our kidneys and zhi will be unfavorably affected, which will require freeing these blockages. Treatment and cultivation to allow expression of this aspect of life can enable a person to live from their Shen.

The kidneys open to the ears. Zhi imbalances can manifest in hearing conditions, not only diminished hearing, but also not hearing or understanding what others are saying.

The liver (hun)

The liver houses the hun, which corresponds to the ethereal shen. The hun relates to the collective consciousness. It is the "we" aspect of consciousness or awareness. A person with a wood/hun imbalance can be driven by the need to be active in working with others for the benefit of the community, society or the collective; the person is compensating for a lack of this area in their life. This activity or expression can include putting oneself in situations that allow concerns for others to manifest, which helps raise awareness of this situation and the opportunity to learn about it and grow. If a person has been in an environment that blocks this expression, they may act in a way that is contrary to their desired behavior (the person is not able to live in a natural way; a suppressed or repressed blockage is preventing this expression). This might be acting in a selfish way, which is the opposite of unity and community. A treatment plan for this person would be to unblock the areas of stagnation to allow expression related to the hun.

Balance is key in Chinese medicine. Our Shen temperament needs to be balanced. If one's expression is extreme, it is not balanced and can lead to pathological patterns. If hun qualities are expressed to an extreme, one can be too attached to the collective and other people, to the cost of one's own health and well-being. In a way, a person may be rejecting their life and taking on the extreme wood nature of rising and flying away, which can be an escape from their body or their life. Balanced activity is a key to creating an environment for personal development.

The liver and hun relate to planning and thinking of the future and how to achieve goals. If there is an extreme or imbalanced quality within these aspects of a person, we can consider it a hun imbalance and condition. We can develop a treatment plan to clear the blockages in the channels and the organs and let a normal flow of energy through the liver and the entire body. This normal flow of qi, which includes the psycho-emotional condition, contributes to restoring balance.

The liver opens to the eyes. Hun imbalances can manifest in seeing problems, diminished eyesight or lack of perception. This can be a lack of insight or inner seeing, not just physical vision.

The lungs (po)

The lungs house the po, which corresponds to the corporeal shen. The po relates to the physical body. The correspondences include the senses, desires and pleasure. Imbalances in the po can manifest as over-attachments to those areas of life. The po can be expressed as selfishness. It's the "me, me, me" aspect of self. Selfishness and greediness can be part of a po disharmony.

The large intestine is the only primary channel that crosses the midline of the body. Some refer to it as the channel of polarity. A polarized po is a common condition in modern society. Loneliness is a common condition of the imbalanced po. Part of this comes from its ability to polarize itself, causing separation from others, society and life itself. Out of this polarity, isolation, separation and an intensified loneliness can occur. These imbalanced experiences and emotions can prompt a response to the polarization, which can initiate change. Loneliness and unhappiness can lead a person to seek another way to live and experience life; the driving force is the body's innate intelligence to seek balance. The practitioner can develop a treatment plan to release the intensities of an imbalanced po. The treatment can include a luo mai treatment to release the emotions, and a divergent channel treatment on the lungs and large intestine channels can assist in the release.

The lungs are connected to the nose. Breathing is a key to bringing the po into the present moment, freeing one from the polarity of the po. There is no polarity or separation in the present moment. Polarity only occurs in thoughts of the past or the future. Polarity creates separation, isolation and loneliness. Breathing practices, including qi gong and tai chi chuan, are traditional ways to regulate the breath, calm the po and promote balance.

The spleen (yi)

The spleen houses the yi shen. The yi corresponds to intellect, thoughts, concepts, ideas and beliefs. The element of the spleen is earth. Grounding, organizing and digestion are qualities of the earth, the spleen and the stomach. The spleen corresponds to the mouth, which processes food and drink and transforms them into nutritive substances. The condition of the spleen and the stomach directly influences that transformation process. Transforming food and drink is the physical transformation. The earth organs, the spleen and stomach, are also involved in the psycho-emotional transformation process. Similar to how food and drink go into the mouth to be processed and transformed, all experiences in life are processed by the yi. The yi processes our life experiences; it organizes, categorizes, filters and makes sense of experiences. In the same way that the condition of the spleen and the stomach determines the quality of the nutrition processed from digesting food, the condition of the yi is instrumental in the processing of our experiences in life, as well as our emotional well-being.

The condition of our yi, which includes the way we perceive, experience and process life, influences the hun, po, zhi and shen. The yi includes our thinking and opinions about people and life. If the yi is in an imbalanced or unhealthy state, all the five shen and their correspondences are influenced. The yi, as the transformer, processes our experiences. The yi includes the intellect and thoughts. When these qualities are over-developed, the other aspects of our body, mind and spirit become imbalanced. When the yi is imbalanced, we become rigid and narrow and respond to life in a conditioned way. We often respond to life based on our past experiences. However, often the past understanding is rooted in fear, anger, misconceptions and prejudice; these influences create a conditioned response.

The yi is susceptible to fixed, rigid and repetitive patterns and reactions based on past experiences. One reason is that the spleen, and therefore the yi, has a function of holding. The spleen holds blood in the vessels; the yi holds as well. It holds emotions and thoughts in the mind and in the blood. This holding function explains how the yi holds onto experiences and how we can live in these held experiences; this is living in the past.

The yi includes mindfulness. What we place attention on and retain in our mind is mindfulness. The yi can be overwhelmed by experiences, especially when we are at a young age and not capable of dealing with them. The yi can go into survival mode and create patterns of behavior that can become constitutional—reactive ways of responding to life. These imprints need to be understood so that we can be released from their influence. When we do that we can be open to the spontaneity of life. Becoming open to life as it is, not what it should be, not what it must be and not as we desire it to be, allows us to live from our Shen. Living from our Shen allows us to live in the present moment and in a spontaneous way.

The yi can be imbalanced when one is too attached to thoughts and emotions. A person can become trapped in them. Then they are living in past experiences. They can also be worrying about the future; in this case they are living in the future. A person will tend to suffer from repetitive and obsessive thoughts and thinking due to the inability to let go. Not being able to let go prevents one from living in the present moment. Feelings can be viewed as normal, natural aspects of life. And they are spontaneous. An imbalanced yi can try to hold onto these feelings, trying to artificially retain something that should be experienced and allowed to leave, like the way the sun and the moon flow through endless cycles of waxing and waning. This *trying* creates a separation that blocks us from fully experiencing the present moment.

The imbalanced yi will hold and maintain past experiences, keeping them alive by continual thinking. Viewing these feelings as *wei* or superficial energetics is Yang. This energetic quality includes the natural flow of appearing and leaving. To keep these feelings alive takes Yin, which has the quality to store and maintain. The spleen and the yi's Yin quality is blood. Through continual thinking about feelings or experiences, the spleen's energetics transform them into emotions, which are then stored in the blood. This process illustrates how we keep emotions alive. What we hold is not the real experience, it is a thought or memory. This holding process becomes part of conditioning and eventually it can become part of the constitution. It can lead to the inability to live in a spontaneous way.

The yi corresponds to earth, which has the qualities of being rooted and grounded. The yi also includes the stomach and spleen's innate quality of being grounded in one's thoughts. Being stuck in one's thoughts can prevent a person from being open to new viewpoints, understandings, choices and actions. This stagnation prevents us from letting go of the past, preventing the ability to experience life in a spontaneous way. Dampness and phlegm can manifest from these stagnations, creating blockages and a rigidity against seeing new things in life. Damp and phlegm can be viewed as the physical manifestation of concepts and thoughts that slow us down and stagnate us.

The spleen opens to the mouth. Yi imbalances can manifest in eating disorders because imbalances of the spleen/stomach and the yi/mouth can be expressed in the mouth and eating.

In my experience, the yi is the main cause of emotional conditions. How the yi is involved in the creation of emotions is explained in the next chapter.

Summary

Imbalances of the five shen, especially the emotions, can transfer to the organs, all the channels and the luo mai. For example, anger can influence the muscle channels, which influences posture and the musculo-skeletal system. Anger can be held in the luo mai, influencing blood. Anger can also influence the main channels and the functions of the organs. It is common for anger to influence digestion. This is wood overacting on earth. Anger can transfer into the divergent channels, causing stagnations and pain in those channels. And when anger becomes an ongoing and chronic experience, it can enter the eight extraordinary channels and become part of the constitution. The process of the emotion anger transferring to other channel systems reflects the interdependent nature of the channel system.

The luo mai can clear pathogenic factors that can cause or exacerbate psycho-emotional imbalances. Making a diagnosis based on the five shen provides a targeted model for treatment. A luo mai treatment is an effective way to release emotionally charged (active) energy.

When treating suppressed and latent pathogens, it may be necessary to release them with treatments that include the eight extraordinary channels, the divergent channels and the main channels to bring them to the surface of the body. When they reach the superficial layer of the body, which is the area where the luo mai are located, a luo mai treatment can release them from the body. With this type of treatment the patient generally feels immediate relief. Lifestyle guidance is often part of the treatment plan, which may include seeing a professional therapist and medical physician. Having the patient perform the healing sounds at home is a fantastic form of daily practice for them that supports a luo mai treatment. A daily practice is a key to change.

FIVE SHEN GROUP DYNAMICS

The five shen is a model that can become the basis of diagnosis and treatment plans. When the five shen correspondences become familiar, their imbalances become clear. The root of an imbalance can originate from a variety of sources, including prenatal and postnatal influences.

It is important to view the five shen as five aspects of one Shen (a person). Each of the five shen contains unique aspects of a person. And each shen shapes other shen in a way required for a person to be whole. The five phases cycles illustrate important relationships within the five shen. Figure 6.2 depicts the five shen in circular formation. When the controlling (ko) cycle is in balance, it is a harmonizing force. When there is an imbalance it can create unfavorable conditions; it can be overacting. The organs/shen contain an innate intelligence, which contains a message to be sent to its related shen (it provides an integral aspect of the functioning of its partner). The five phases cycles are the patterns for these integral relationships.

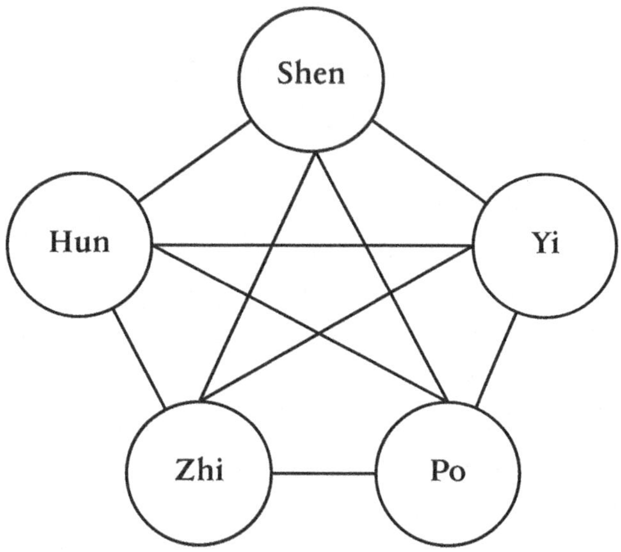

Figure 6.2 The five shen

The five shen (five phases) cycles contain a shaping or message-sharing function. For example, the heart shen or fire has a controlling or shaping relationship with the lungs and the po. The heart shen sends its energy or message to the po. The message from the heart shen to the lung po is that we are essentially spirit. This realization guides the po spirit in its expression of the physical aspect of life. The po qualities are close to the physical body, the physical aspect of life. When it is imbalanced it is susceptible to being polarized, creating imbalances that can manifest as selfishness. This selfishness can include an unhealthy pursuit of one's own needs, desires and pleasures, often ignoring other people's needs. It's the heart shen that expresses to the po its original nature, the yuan shen. The balance of the two allows for the smooth expression of po in life. This expression is guided by the heart shen. When the shen and the po are in balance, this interaction and exchange is always occurring. When we create a life that maintains this relationship, our experience is a natural, spontaneous expression of spirit. It can be called living in the Tao, or living in spirit. Spiritual traditions around the world call it Christ consciousness, Krishna consciousness or Buddha nature.

The po and hun

The po shen contains the innate intelligence of the importance of living in this world, enjoying it and allowing full expression of our life in the here and now. The po sends this message to the hun spirit (metal controlling or shaping wood), which is the ethereal spirit. The hun includes the collective aspect of our life. This is the aspect of our life that we experience when we are attuned to the whole, part of a collective society and a unified universe.

When the hun is imbalanced it can include a denial of the physical body; this can be when a person pursues a spiritual direction in an attempt to deny the physical body and life. If there is a rejection of the physical body and life, a deep polarization can occur. The imbalanced hun can cause an individual to be too involved in society or assisting others to the detriment of their own health. One may believe it is of greater value to help others, but if it is a denial of a healthy enjoyment of their physical life and body then it is a rejection of their physical needs and desires. This rejection can create a polarity and separation, which creates an imbalance not only of the po and hun, but also of the other shen. The po–hun relationship includes the balanced relationship between self and others, and the individual and society.

The hun and yi

The hun contains the innate intelligence of the collective aspect of life. The hun sends this message to the yi, the spleen's shen. This interaction is wood shaping or influencing earth. The yi contains our conceptual or intellectual capabilities. This is our ability to reason, be logical and organize and categorize; it includes intention (focus). The spleen and the yi process not only food and drink but also our experiences of life. When the yi is imbalanced it can lead to separation of oneself from other people and society, creating isolation and polarization.

Being too attached to thoughts and concepts turns a person's attention from real life, which creates a schism, because the body innately knows there is one reality. The reality is living in the present. Additionally, an imbalanced yi can manifest as obsessive and repetitive actions. These actions may be rooted in an extreme or distorted understanding or perception of experiences or thoughts. The hun can send its energy and message to the yi: the message is that we are part of the whole of life, not separate from it. Yi qualities are just one aspect of a person and not the primary aspect. The hun can help balance the yi to receive and process life in a clear, spontaneous way, and not in a conditioned, repetitive way.

The yi and zhi

The yi or earth shapes or sends a message to the zhi, the shen of the kidneys. The zhi contains an innate intelligence of our unlimited nature, the capacity to become anything: this is called "chaos" in Taoist philosophy; it is our primordial nature. It is before thinking, before the dualistic categorization of all things in life. When the yi aspect of our life is over-developed, we become conditioned in how we respond to people, activities and situations. An imbalanced yi can have a significant influence on the zhi. It can overact on it, forcing it into a specific shape, which can prevent its natural freeflowing nature from being expressed.

The zhi contains willpower, the will and power to achieve goals and objectives. It is also the will and power to live the type of life we desire. One variation of this is the will and desire to seek our true nature, and then live from it. Zhi corresponds to water. Water's nature includes taking any form or shape; it is the flexibility to adapt to all situations. The zhi loathes cold. One reason for this is that cold freezes water, changing its innate nature of adaptability. The yi can help shape the zhi to accomplish goals and objectives. One way it does this is by applying *focus* on achieving or accomplishing.

The zhi needs some direction or focus, or it can spread itself too much and not accomplish what it wants. The relationship between the yi and the zhi, earth and water, and the prenatal and postnatal, can be found in many aspects of Chinese medicine. One interesting relationship is between the Chong channel and the spleen and stomach. The Chong channel, which originates in the uterus and kidneys, flows to qi chong, Stomach 30. The stomach channel is earth, and this pathway connection illustrates earth shaping the form of jing as it unfolds in life. Additionally, gongsun, Spleen 4, is the opening point of the chong channel; this relationship is also earth shaping water. It is the postnatal shaping prenatal.

A balanced yi provides a favorable focus and intention that allows the zhi to unfold in a healthy way. If the yi is imbalanced it can cause rigid thinking and actions, and can create repetitive and obsessive activities. The zhi needs the yi to have an openness to receive and experience life. Openness allows the zhi to maintain the ability to be flexible and adaptive. The zhi needs this to allow its natural unfolding and the fulfillment of one's destiny.

The zhi and shen

The zhi or water shapes and sends its energy to the heart shen. This relationship is the classic Chinese model of Yin–Yang, water–fire, Shao Yin and Jing–Shen. This relationship can be viewed as the zhi's capacity to become anything. There is a clear direction within all these possibilities: it is Jing seeking Shen, the zhi seeking the heart shen. The kidneys' external pathway, the pathway where the points are located, flows past the heart area and contains the front shu points. These five points have a profound influence on the five shen. The points are presented in Chapter 58 of the *Su Wen*, "The Acupuncture Points."

The heart shen contains our true nature. Some traditions view realization of this aspect of our nature as the primary goal or purpose of life. This realization provides the opportunity to live from this awareness. Jing seeking shen can be viewed as our quest in life. The models of Jing–Shen, water–fire and Yin–Yang, along with the trajectory connections between the kidneys and heart, show the inner energetic system reflecting this quest.

Table 6.1 summarizes fundamental information about the five shen. This information can be used to make a five shen diagnosis.

Table 6.1 Five shen and correspondences

Zhi Water	Kidneys Bladder	Lineage, genetics, willpower, reproduction, vision, dreams, destiny, unlimited possibilities, destiny code, the will to live your destiny
Hun Wood	Liver Gallbladder	Collective, intelligence, growth, cultivation, direction, ethereal, planning, decision making, judgments
Shen Fire	Heart Small Intestine	Spirit, consciousness, quest, guidance, intuition, wisdom, yuan shen, true spirit
Yi Earth	Spleen Stomach	Concepts, thoughts, intellect, grounding, rooting, practical, digesting life experiences, organizing, holding emotions/thoughts/blood, mindfulness, polarity, separation
Po Metal	Lungs Large Intestine	Physical body, physical desires, sensitivity to emotions, selfishness, isolation, inability to forgive

CHAPTER 7

THE EMOTIONS

The early practitioners of Chinese medicine had a profound understanding of how the psycho-emotional condition of a person can influence that person's life. They understood the inseparable relationship between the physical body and emotions. The Han dynasty classic, the *Nei Jing*, presents the six exogenous pathogens (wind, cold, damp, heat, summer heat and dryness) and the seven emotions as major causes of illness. The seven emotions are anger, joy, sadness, grief, pensiveness, fear and fright. These practitioners perceived that the emotions and the organs (physical body) influence each other. The understanding of this symbiotic relationship is the basis of holistic healing and Chinese medicine.

The ancient healers differentiated natural virtues and emotions. Natural virtues occur when we live in a natural and spontaneous way. The natural virtues are the fundamental qualities of a person. In the Taoist tradition of Lao Zi, Wu Wei ("nothing extra") is the name given to the natural and spontaneous way of living life. The Taoists experienced how living in Wu Wei naturally attuned a person to their Shen, and allowed their life to be an expression of it. The natural expression includes living in balance. Balance encompasses a range, not a point. Within this view of balance is the ability to respond to situations in an appropriate way, which at times can create an imbalance, following which one naturally adjusts back to a balanced state. The adjusting is the key. If a person has clarity about who they are, in this case their Shen (Shen is the natural self), they are able to deal with difficulties and challenges in life from their Shen, and if they are thrown off balance they will realign to their natural self. The duration of this realigning process varies amongst people. With a clear understanding of what we are (Shen), the duration decreases; one reason for this is release from attachments to a false identity. The incorrect belief about what someone thinks or feels they are is diminished, and in some cases eliminated. Being free from this veil of false identity allows awareness of their Shen, and the opportunity to be a living expression of Shen in their normal, everyday life. A common way to describe this is "present-awareness." In my experience, being mindful of present-awareness is living in Wu Wei.

WHAT ARE EMOTIONS?

From a Taoist psychological viewpoint, emotions can be described as an experience that creates a psycho-emotional imbalance strong enough that a person does not live from balance and naturalness. Emotions are a normal part of life. A goal is to be able to let them go and not retain them for longer than a normal time frame. A normal time frame can vary for each person. Most spiritual traditions include forgiveness and unconditional love as part of their value system; both are a way of letting go. Letting go of emotions and imbalanced experiences allows for experiencing the present moment and its spontaneity. The ancient healers created numerous ways that can help let go of experiences and emotions that create imbalances. Qi gong, meditation, reading, chanting, herbal medicine, acupuncture and *I Ching* and *Tao Teh Ching* philosophy are some of the methods and philosophies that comprise cultivation practices for understanding life stresses and the imbalances they can create. Luo mai treatments can assist in the letting go of emotional qi. *Prick to bleed* is a way to release emotional qi. A prick to bleed luo mai treatment can assist a person in adjusting to their natural self.

Emotions are a major cause of illness and changes in the disposition of a person. As a major cause of imbalance it is necessary to understand what they are, how they are formed and how they can be treated. Emotions have a strong effect on the heart and the Shen. In Chinese medicine, the heart is the residence of the Shen. Chapter 71 of the *Ling Shu*, "The Evil Guest," presents this relationship.

> Qi Bo said, "The heart is the grand master of the five organs and the six bowels. The heart is the shelter of seminal essence and spirit.

> The organs are solid. Evil must not appear. If it appears it causes injury to the heart and the spirit to depart, which causes death."[25]

This *Ling Shu* reference can be interpreted as saying that the heart is the grand master (the center of importance and influence) of the internal organs and their correspondences. These correspondences include the natural virtues and emotions. Evil pathogenic factors (exogenous and endogenous pathogenic factors) must not enter the heart because if the heart is injured, then the internal organs, Jing and the Shen will be harmed. If the heart is injured, the spirit will depart and this will cause death. "Death" can mean that a person feels separate, alone, lost and isolated (socially isolated). In this instance, the injured heart causes a polarity and a feeling of separation. The polarity, separation, isolation and the feeling of being lost influence the entire person. The seminal essence is Jing, and it represents both the physical body and the psycho-emotional condition generated by life experiences. These experiences are held in the body (Jing), creating imprints and conditioning; this is a normal process. It is these life experiences that are harming the balance within the five shen and Shen awareness; and *attachment to the yi* (the imbalances) is part of this conditioning. The attachment is part of the holding. If the heart and Shen are harmed, the body and mind are affected. Having a healthy heart and Shen is essential for having a healthy life. The *Ling Shu* passage quoted above reminds us of this reality of life.

The *Su Wen* and the *Ling Shu* describe how pathogens can transfer throughout the body. The six exogenous pathogenic factors can be transferred from the superficial levels to the deeper levels of the body. The seven emotions (emotional qi) can be transferred into the blood, muscles, acupuncture channels and internal organs. They can also enter the deep Jing levels to become part of the constitution. This transfer is part of the process by means of which emotions can influence the entire body and how they are held in the body. The yi plays an essential role in holding emotions in the body.

HOW EMOTIONS ARE FORMED

Human life includes a wide range of experiences. As we interact in life and accumulate experiences, we process them. The processing of experiences includes making sense of them, which contributes to the formation of the ego. The ego is part of the yi. The choices we make in our daily life are influenced by the yi. All being well, a nurturing, supporting and loving environment is provided during early childhood to allow natural and healthy interactions for development of the yi. When that environment does not exist, a process of emotional pathology can occur. The repetitive influences of an unhealthy environment create a conditioning and a powerful influence on a person. The ancient healers understood this process and developed ways to assist a person in changing the effects of it. Part of this change involves understanding how imbalanced emotions are formed.

THE FORMATION OF THE YI

The formation of the yi involves life interactions and their influences in our life. If there is a loving and encouraging environment, a child is influenced by it. How does this influence occur? It is by daily exposure that influences all layers of a person: the physical, mental/emotional and the spiritual. All "three treasures" are influenced by it. This continual influence can form a healthy yi that enters the Jing level and becomes the constitution and the fundamental aspect of a person. If, by contrast, a child is in an environment that is continually full of anger, fear, sadness, depression and worry, they continually feel them and the feelings enter the child's deep levels (Jing; eight extraordinary channels).

When a child is continually exposed to either of these environments, the experiences become part of the yi. An analogy would be how the quality of the food and fluids we consume each day influences our body and mind. Years and decades of a certain nutritional quality profoundly influence a person. If the nutritional quality is good, there is a good influence. If it is not good, there is an unfavorable influence on health. This process works the same way in the emotional environment (the yi digesting and processing life experiences). We can view emotions as emotional qi, and this qi is continually influencing Jing–Qi–Shen (body–mind–spirit).

When each person is living a natural and spontaneous life, the natural virtues are expressed spontaneously. When we live from a conditioned response, we are living from deep, old patterns of experiences. We are not living in the present, but living from memories of the past or dreams of the future. Emotions can become the basis of conditioned responses to life. For example, when a child is around an angry person every day, there is a good chance that they are being influenced by that emotion. They can express anger in the way they act, regardless of whether it is an appropriate response to a situation. The person can also repress anger, causing anger qi to flow deeper in the channel system, the internal organs and Jing. The emotion is internalized. This can cause a powerful effect on the liver and gallbladder organs and their correspondences. Because the five phases influence each other, this influence can influence other organs. For example, the hun can influence its child, the shen; its grandchild, the yi; the grandparent, the po; and its parent, the zhi.

Chapter 62 of the *Su Wen*, "Regulation of the Channels," says the following about the five shen.

> The five types of excess and deficiency are borne from the five zang organs. For example, the heart houses the shen or spirit; the lungs house the qi; the liver accommodates the blood; the spleen houses the form and flesh; and the kidneys house the zhi, or will. They must all function together as the zhi and the shen are functioning in concert psychically, connecting with the bones and marrow within and forming the shape of the body without. This creates an entire functioning being and is the makeup of the human body. Within the five zang, communication occurs via pathways or channels, which transport qi and blood. When the qi and blood are not regulated, illness occurs. Diagnosis and treatment depend on channels and pathways.[26]

This passage from the *Su Wen* describes how the proper functioning of the five zang organs and the circulation of qi and blood is necessary for health. Emotions can unfavorably influence both of those functions, causing, in turn, an unfavorable influence on the Shen. Maintaining a healthy emotional condition is essential for health and vitality.

A key to health, vitality and well-being is a healthy circulation of qi and blood throughout the body. Qi comprises everything in life. It encompasses feelings, emotions and experiences. If the emotions create a stagnation and blockage, they can create illness of the body–mind–spirit (Jing–Qi–Shen). Medical practitioners should be able to determine where these stagnations exist. The framework for determining where stagnation exists can be the channel system: the muscle, luo, main, divergent and/or the eight extraordinary channels and collaterals. Identifying the channels involved provides the basis for a targeted treatment. Emotional stagnations can influence all the channel systems and the internal organs. Understanding the process of how the environment and lifestyle influence a person offers a way to reverse the influence. Chinese medicine, medical qi gong and lifestyle guidance, along with the appropriate allopathic medical care, can assist a person in changing their life.

CHINESE MEDICAL THEORY OF BLOOD AND EMOTIONS

The creation of blood

In Chinese medicine, food and fluids are transformed and transported in the spleen and the stomach. One transformation of these substances is into gu qi, which is transported to the lungs and the heart to eventually create blood. The heart then circulates the blood throughout the body. The spleen assists the heart in the circulation of blood by holding it in the blood vessels. The focus in this section is the relationship between the spleen, the heart and blood; other organs are involved in the creation of blood but their relationships are not discussed in this chapter.

Creating, circulating and holding blood in the blood vessels are the three main functions of the spleen and the heart. *Understanding these functions contributes to understanding the formation and holding of emotions in the body.* They also provide a framework for developing treatment plans.

The Shen and blood

In Chinese medicine the heart houses the Shen, and the Shen's qualities include our emotional well-being. The heart is also involved in the creation and circulation of blood. Those three functions of the heart—housing the Shen, and making and circulating blood—link the heart, the Shen, emotions and blood. This dynamic explains one aspect of why the Shen and emotions are stored in the blood.

The spleen and blood

The spleen works with the heart to make and circulate blood. The spleen creates gu qi from food and fluids, and sends it to the lungs and the heart to make blood. The spleen's energetics include holding blood in the vessels. When it does not hold blood in the vessels, there can be reckless bleeding. This is the spleen's physical function.

There is also a psycho-emotional holding. The yi holds thoughts, feelings, emotions and experiences in the blood. When the yi does not hold and release in a balanced way, it can cause reckless mental activity. When the yi holds too much, there can be repetitive and possibly obsessive thinking.

The yi and the ego

The spleen holds physical substances, thoughts and emotions. The yi, the spleen's shen, embraces our intellectual, conceptual and thinking qualities. It includes our ego. The formation of our ego, opinions, preferences and emotional attachments is part of the yi. While the spleen holds blood in the vessels, the yi holds thoughts, feelings and emotions in the blood. The spleen holds all of its correspondences. This physical and psycho-emotional function explains how the spleen and thoughts, feelings and emotions are stored in the blood.

When we do not let go of emotions (experiences), the body can respond in several ways. First, emotions are qi. Qi is Yang compared to blood, which is Yin. The emotion (Yang) is stored in a Yin substance, blood. When there is repetitive thinking, the body believes the person wants to keep these thoughts and the feelings associated with them. The heart and the spleen will hold them in the blood, the Yin substance related to these organs. The body will assist in the desire to hold the experiences. This is the yi function of holding. When we have experiences and want to maintain it and relive them, or when we have trauma and can't let go of it, all of the five shen and the Shen can be influenced as a result of the yi becoming overly active in its inability to let go of the experience and the emotion(s). In other words, the yi holds onto the experiences and continually relives them; this is the holding function. We then live from this past experience, or from a desire for something to manifest in the future. This creates a pattern or imprint that is repeated until the experience is let go and the natural virtues within a person can be expressed.

HOW EMOTIONS CAN INFLUENCE A PERSON

Each day and night, blood circulates throughout the entire body. During this circulation the qualities in the blood, which include emotions, continually influence a person. Initially this influence is at a superficial level, but if the circulation of emotional qi continues it will eventually enter the deeper levels of a person. The influence flows from the wei level to the yuan level. (Trauma can enter the yuan level quickly.) This process indicates how important it is to let go of emotions to maintain a healthy psycho-emotional condition. The *Su Wen* and the *Ling Shu* describe numerous ways in which pathogens can transfer through the body. For example, in Chapter 63 of the *Su Wen*, "Acupuncturing the Superficial Luo," pathogens in the luo collaterals can transfer first to the main channels and then to the internal organs. Also, the Ying Qi cycle (daily clock), which is described in Chapter 16 of the *Ling Shu*, "Nourishing Qi," suggests that postnatal pathogens can move through the body from the lungs to the liver. In this cycle, not only does the cycle flow back to the lungs from the liver to repeat an endless process through the 12 channels, the internal organs and the five shen, but a branch also flows to the Du and the Ren channels. This connection from the main channels to the eight extraordinary channels is a reminder that if we do not resolve issues in our daily life, they can move deeper into the constitutional level.

The process of emotionally charged blood circulating throughout the body influencing Jing, Qi and Shen also explains the process whereby emotions can influence our well-being and health. There is a way to use this process to circulate natural virtues to rejuvenate the body. With qi gong, meditation, prayer, reading, etc., we can fill the yi with the natural virtues and enlightening experiences. With continual practice (cultivation) the yi holds them in thoughts (mindfulness) and eventually in our blood. These natural experiences and virtues will circulate throughout the body to nourish it. The effects will flow from the wei level to the yuan level. This is a way to change our life. The "six healing sounds" is a powerful way to begin that process.

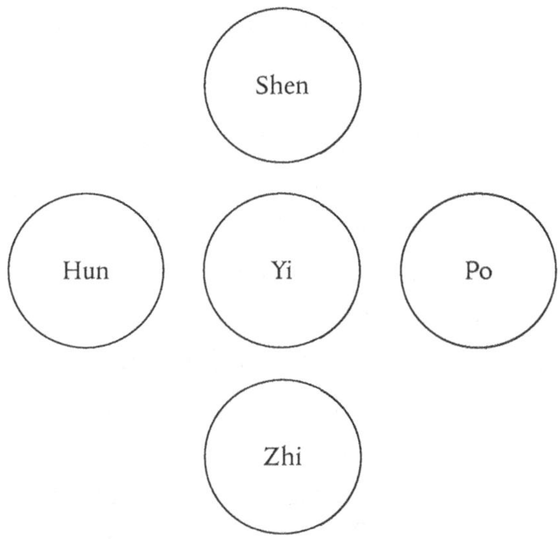

Figure 7.1 The yi shen as the center and transformer

The yi is the filtering mechanism of life experiences (Figure 7.1). If we change the yi, we change our ability to experience life. Treating emotions in the blood can release the intensity of the emotion. It is a powerful way of letting them go. It is a physical letting go that influences our psycho-emotional condition as the blood is released from the body (prick to bleed method), and with it goes the emotionally charged energy.

THE LUO MAI AND BLOOD

In the acupuncture channel system the luo collaterals include pathways of blood. The early Chinese medical practitioners described the different luo mai. There are the major luo mai, which are the traditional pathways presented in the *Ling Shu*. There are also the smaller luo mai, which are listed below.

1. *Bie luo.* These are the large luo mai. Bie luo are collaterals that divert or branch off the main channel. They are the major luo.

2. *Fu luo.* They are the floating or superficial luo. They are the blood vessels that are visible.

3. *Sun luo.* These are the grandchild or descendant luo. They are minute (tiny) collaterals (small sub-branches) and are a couple of generations down from the bie luo.

When treating the luo collaterals, the blood is treated. The classical method of treatment is pricking (bloodletting) with a lancet or other pricking device. A goal is to remove the pathogen in the blood from the body. Bloodletting removes the blood from the body. This is a form of letting go. Because the luo collaterals treat blood they have an influence on the *correspondences* of blood, which include the heart, the heart shen, the yi and emotions. This relationship is one explanation for why the luo collaterals can treat the Shen and psycho-emotional conditions.

The heart is considered the location of the Shen. It is both the central Shen from a one-Shen perspective, and it is the heart shen from a five-shen perspective. Every emotional condition that reaches an imbalanced state can influence the heart shen. The more polarized and extreme the emotion, the more powerful the effect it has on the Shen. This dynamic is similar to all insomnia involving the heart. The five shen are really one Shen; they are five aspects of the one Shen. Therefore, any emotional condition can influence the heart and the Shen.

Treating only the luo collaterals with bloodletting is not enough to treat long-term psycho-emotional patterns and conditioning. Treating the yi is an essential part of a treatment plan. Strategies can include treating the eight extraordinary channels, the divergent channels and the primary channels to influence the long-term conditioning. Treating the luo collaterals can provide quick relief and an outlet for acute emotional conditions. It can also be part of a treatment that is designed to bring chronic and repressed emotional qi to the surface and then release it. Releasing pathogenic factors (in this case the emotions) is a main function of the luo collaterals.

Chapter 8

WINDOW OF THE SKY POINTS

The acupuncture point category *window of the sky points* is a modern creation. Using these points to obtain spiritual insight or guidance is also a modern creation. There is no reference in Chinese medical texts for an acupuncture point category called "window of the sky." The history of this category of points is very interesting. Chapter 21 of the *Ling Shu*, "Cold and Hot Diseases," presents a variety of points that treat a variety of conditions including muscular pain, rheumatism and conditions of the face and neck. There are five points listed together in one paragraph, and in the following paragraph the conditions they treat are listed. There is no group or category name for the five points, and the chapter presents only five points, not the ten that are commonly presented nowadays as the window of the sky points. The classical function of these five points is basically treating the imbalanced flow of qi and blood. The following summarizes the function of each of the five points.

- **Man's Receptor—Ren Ying—Stomach 9:** When Yang is rebellious and there is counterflow, there is pain in the head. The chest is full and one is unable to take breath normally. For this condition treat Man's Receptor.
- **Supporting Chimney—Fu Tu—Large Intestine 18:** When there is abrupt loss of speech, the qi hardens; treat Supporting Chimney.
- **Celestial Pillar—Tian You—San Jiao 16:** When there is abrupt loss of hearing, the qi becomes covered and blocked, and the ears and eyes lose their brightness; treat Celestial Pillar.

- **Wind Pillar—Tian Zhu—Bladder 10:** When there are spasms, convulsions and dizziness, and the feet are unable to bear the body, treat Wind Pillar.
- **Celestial Mansion—Tian Fu—Lung 3:** An abrupt thirst and fever, the interior is rebellious and in counterflow, causing the liver and lungs to strike at each other, and blood overflows from the nose and mouth; treat Celestial Mansion.

Additionally, the paragraph ends with the following sentence: "The five points for treatment include San Jiao 16, Tian You (celestial/sky window), and its surrounding points."[27]

There is no name or function for this group of five points. The earliest reference to it as window of the sky points appears to be from Dr. Albert Chamfrault. The name "window of the sky" appeared in print in 1954, in Dr. Chamfrault's book *Traité de Médecine Chinoise, Tome 1: Acupuncture, Moxas, Massages, Saignées.* San Jiao 16, Tian You (celestial/sky window), was most likely based on the sentence quoted above.

Dr. Chamfrault calls the five points in Chapter 21 of the *Ling Shu* the "big window of the sky" points. Dr. Nguyen Van Nghi uses the name "five great windows of heaven" (Tian Wu Bu) for the same five points, in his translation of Chapter 21 of the *Ling Shu.* Dr. Nghi states that "the five great windows" cited in the previous chapter are grouped under the name Tian You Wu Bu (group of five great windows of the heaven).[28]

THE TEN POINTS

In Chapter 2 of the *Ling Shu,* "The Roots of the Acupuncture Points," certain acupuncture points along the main channels, as well as regions of the body, are presented. One of the regions contains the following ten points:

> In the middle of the body between the Broken Dish (supraclavicular fossae) is the Conception Vessel. This point is called **Celestial Chimney**. On the first line following the sides of the Conception Vessel are beating pulses (carotid pulses) on the Leg Bright Yang at points called **Man's Receptor**. The second line from the channel of the Conception Vessel is the Arm Bright Yang at points called

> **Supporting Chimney**. The third line from the channel is the Arm Major Yang with points called **Celestial Window**. The fourth line from the channel is the Arm Minor Yang at points called **Celestial Shutters**. The sixth line from the channel is the Leg Major Yang at points called **Celestial Pillar**. The seventh line from the channel is on the Governing Vessel Channel right through the middle of the neck. The point is called **Wind Pillar**. On the further side of it is the point **Wind Mansion**. In the fossa of the armpit is a beating pulse on the Arm Major Yin. This point is called **Celestial Mansion**. Below the armpit by three cun is the Arm Pericardium Channel. This point is called Tian Chi, **Celestial Pool**.[29]

These ten points are listed in Table 8.1.

Table 8.1 The ten points (window of the sky points)

English name	Acupoint	Pin Yin name
Celestial Chimney	Ren 22	Tian Tu
Man's Receptor/ Prognosis	Stomach 9	Ren Ying*
Supporting Chimney	Large Intestine 18	Fu Tu*
Celestial Window	Small Intestine 16	Tian Chuang
Celestial Shutters/ Appearance	Small Intestine 17	Tian Rong
Celestial Pillar/ Window	San Jiao 16	Tian You*
Wind Pillar/Celestial Pillar	Bladder 10	Tian Zhu*
Wind Mansion	Du 16	Feng Fu
Celestial Mansion/ Storehouse	Lung 3	Tian Fu*
Celestial Pool	Pericardium 1	Tian Chi

* *Included among the five points listed in Chapter 21 of the Ling Shu.*

Dr. Chamfrault and Dr. Nghi collaborated in naming the additional five points listed in Chapter 2 of the *Ling Shu* the "little window of the sky" points.

Eventually, all ten came to be called collectively the window of the sky points. Word of this new group of points and their new functions (receiving guidance, inspiration and insights from the celestial/heaven) spread around the world. Everyone who now teaches and uses these ten points as the window of the sky points is following the work of Chamfrault and Nghi. This acupuncture group is not based on any Chinese medical source.

TWICKEN'S THEORY OF THE WINDOW OF THE SKY POINTS

In an effort to understand how the window of the sky points might treat emotional conditions, I have researched the *Su Wen* and the *Ling Shu* for connections with the treatment of emotions. There are two main chapters that present a relationship between the five big window of the sky points and luo points: based on the understanding that the luo points treat emotions, Chapters 2 and 5 of the *Ling Shu* draw connections between luo points and some of the window points.

In Chapter 5 of the *Ling Shu*, "Roots and Ends," there is a passage that makes a unique connection between a series of points that includes the luo and the five window points. There are five sets of points on the Yang channels. They include the well, source, river, window and luo points. This set of points can be viewed as connected, as well as having an influence on each other. Guided by the fundamental treatment method of reinforcing and reducing, these points or selected points in each sequence can be reinforced or reduced. If the classical Yin–Yang treatment of channels is applied (which means to reinforce Yin channels and organs to assist their fundamental quality of gathering and storing (reinforcing), and to reduce Yang channels and organs to assist their emptying function (reducing)), these Yang channel points are reduced. Reducing releases pathogens or imbalanced qi.

The patterns of five points end with the window and the luo points. These five Yang luo points can be expanded to include all the luo mai channels and their respective luo points. I have now found a connection that indicates why window of the sky points can treat emotional conditions. The five points around the neck are close to the main vasculature structures that have a strong influence on blood. This sequence of points linking blood to the luo collaterals includes the window and luo points in the five points sequence, and it can be viewed as a direct link between blood, window of the sky points, the luo points and emotional conditions.

There is another link between the window and the luo points. In Chapter 21 of the *Ling Shu* it says: "When there is rheumatism from counterflow, the rebellious qi goes up in counterflow to the abdomen. Treat the luo points on the Yin and Yang channels." Treating rheumatism is a main function of the luo mai. Chapter 21 also presents a relationship between the five points (window of the sky points) and the luo mai. When Chapters 5 and 21 of the *Ling Shu* are combined, a relationship between the luo points and the five points from Chapter 21 is revealed. Extrapolating from the five channels in Chapter 5 to ten channels (excluding the san jiao and the pericardium), a connection is made between the window of the sky points, the luo points and the five shen. This connection of acupuncture points has clinical applications: the window of the sky points can be used with the luo points to release emotional qi. Table 8.2 lists these points.

I have applied this point sequence in clinical practice. I have tried numerous variations of the points, including all five points in a treatment. I have also treated the window of the sky and the luo points only. I have found those two points, along with other points as part of a treatment, to be very effective in treating emotional conditions. The most effective treatments are needling the window of the sky points and plum blossoming the luo point. (Lancet or superficially needling can be applied as well.) This treatment is a powerful releasing treatment.

Table 8.2 The well, source, river, window of the sky and luo points

This point sequence may also be a source for the development of the source and luo point combination.

Channel	Well Root (begins) Finger–toes	Source Passage Wrist–ankle	River Arrival Arm–leg	Window of the sky Neck	Connecting point Mid-leg–mid-arm
Tai Yang	Bladder 67	Bladder 64	Bladder 60	Bladder 10	Bladder 58
Shao Yang	Gallbladder 44	Gallbladder 40	Gallbladder 38	Small Intestine 17	Gallbladder 37
Yang Ming	Stomach 45	Stomach 42	Stomach 41	Stomach 9	Stomach 40
Tai Yang	Small Intestine 1	Small Intestine 4	Small Intestine 5	Small Intestine 16	Small Intestine 7
Shao Yang	San Jiao 1	San Jiao 4	San Jiao 6	San Jiao 16	San Jiao 5
Yang Ming	Large Intestine 1	Large Intestine 4	Large Intestine 5	Large Intestine 18	Large Intestine 6

I hope this chapter inspires discussion and analysis about the window of the sky points. A goal of this chapter has been to learn about the history of these points and how the category name was created. Ultimately, determining whether these points can be used in clinical practice is most important. I hope this chapter contributes toward that goal.

CHAPTER 9

NEW LUO MAI THEORIES AND APPLICATIONS

The *Nei Jing* includes the luo mai as part of the acupuncture channel system. The function and clinical applications of the luo mai are primarily presented in the *Ling Shu*, Chapter 10, "The Main Channels." The main theories and clinical applications of the luo mai and luo points that have become part of the mainstream practice of acupuncture do not appear to be based on the *Ling Shu*, *Su Wen* or other early classics of Chinese medicine. We will explore some of these theories with the goal of identifying the assumptions and guiding principles for the modern applications. A focused analysis of the assumptions of these new applications may guide the reader to determine whether and how to use them in clinical practice.

THE SOURCE AND LUO POINTS ACUPUNCTURE COMBINATION

Treating the source and luo points together is a modern treatment method that is not found in the early classics of acupuncture. Based on my research, historically there have been four main changes in the way the luo points are applied in clinical practice.

Dou Hanqing created the first change when he introduced the command points for the eight extraordinary channels in 1196 AD. Four of the command points are luo points. The functions of these luo points would include treating the eight extraordinary channels. The vital substances associated with the eight extraordinary channels are jing and source qi. Now four luo points can influence source qi.

The second change is found in the *Zhen Jiu Da Cheng* (*The Great Compendium of Acupuncture and Moxibustion*), written by Yang Jizhou in the Ming dynasty.

The third change occurred with George Soulié de Morant, the French practitioner, writer and teacher, and the fourth occurred with Dr. Albert Chamfrault and Dr. Nguyen Van Nghi.

Each of the theories, assumptions and applications will now be evaluated to gain a deeper understanding of them and their relationship to the teachings of the *Ling Shu.*

Dou Hanqing is a famous practitioner and writer from the Jin dynasty (1115–1234). In 1196 he wrote *The Guide of Acupuncture.* Dou is the individual we can trace who presented and promoted the eight command points of the extraordinary channels. He revealed these points around 1196 AD. They are not in any known texts before his work. He left no theory about how they work, or why each point was selected. Four luo points were selected as command points. The luo points are Lung 7 for the Ren channel, San Jiao 5 for the Yang Wei channel, Pericardium 6 for the Yin Wei channel and Spleen 4 for the Chong channel.

Creating this new point category and assigning this function to the four luo points created new conditions the luo points could treat. It radically changed the function of the luo points. The luo points could now treat jing, source qi and conditions of the eight extraordinary channels. It seems that these four points could treat conditions which the source points would classically treat. I believe this new function contributed to the change in how the luo points were subsequently to be used, and to the basis of the source–luo point combination created in the Ming dynasty. Dou was also very involved in chrono-acupuncture.

Xu Feng was a famous doctor in the Ming dynasty (1368–1644). He continued some of the work of Dou Hanqing and promoted what would become the common coupled pairs of the eight extraordinary channels and their corresponding command points: the Ren (Lung 7) and the Yin Qiao (Kidney 6); the Du (Small Intestine 3) and the Yang Qiao (Bladder 62); the Chong (Spleen 4) and the Yin Wei (Pericardium 6); and the Dai (Gallbladder 41) and the Yang Wei (San Jiao 5). There is no strong Chinese medical theory to support these pairings as unique or more clinically effective than other combinations that could fit a diagnosis and treatment plan. Xu was also very involved in chrono-acupuncture.

The *Zhen Jiu Da Cheng* is a collection of writings from the Han to the Ming Dynasties. In 1601 Yang Jizhou finished writing this text. The *Zhen Jiu Da Cheng* is a classic Chinese medical text. It includes information from the classics, as well as from Yang's family tradition and his own insights. This classic book is the main source of the luo and source point combinations. Yang lists each of the luo and source points for the Yin–Yang channels. He lists symptoms and conditions for each channel. It is common when referring to the luo mai to use the name "luo mai" (connecting collaterals) to distinguish them from other channels. Yang does not list the source–luo point combinations as a luo mai treatment. He lists them according to their organ name, which is a way to reference the main channels. Because the main channels connect to the internal organs, treating the main channels can influence the organs. The way Yang names this combination is important: he is saying that this is a treatment for the main channels and the organs. This is not a luo mai treatment.

Yang does not cite any sources for the luo and source point combination. They are not found in any classic texts before the *Zhen Jiu Da Cheng*. Some scholars believe this source–luo combination came from his family tradition or his own discovery. I speculate that he may have based this point combination on the work of Dou Hanqing. As mentioned already in this chapter, Dou assigned four luo points as command points for the eight extraordinary channels. The luo points could influence the eight extraordinary channels, jing and source qi. I suspect that Yang concluded that all the luo points could influence source qi as well, and that he therefore established a new acupuncture point combination, the source and luo points. The changing function of the luo points (from Dou to Yang) begins a series of radical changes in the conditions that the luo points treat. The shift from treating luo mai symptoms and conditions to treating the main channels and the internal organs can be found in the work of these two practitioners and writers. Most interestingly, there is no theory to support their applications. It will be later practitioners and writers who attempt to explain the reasoning for the new functions of the luo mai, and I will evaluate the assumptions made in their theories.

Yang Jizhou includes some of Dou Hanqing's and Xu Feng's works in Volume V of the *Zhen Jiu Da Cheng*. Yang offers little guidance about the clinical method of applying a source–luo combination. He does not state whether to reinforce or reduce the points. He offers no theory to explain how this point combination would work. Morant, and later Chamfrault and Nghi, would offer theories about how this combination would work, which would change the theory and function of the luo mai in Europe and later around the world.

The *Zhen Jiu Da Cheng* includes symptoms that indicate when to use the source and luo points for treatment. Yang defines the method as the host–guest (it is one of a variety of acupuncture point combinations called host–guest). The list of conditions this point combination can treat ranges beyond the conditions listed in the *Ling Shu*. It represents a radical shift in the function of the luo points. Yang does not distinguish between what the luo points treat and what the source points treat, and he does not describe how they support each other or how they function together.

Yang lists some symptoms from the luo mai found in Chapter 10 of the *Ling Shu*. He also adds from the same chapter symptoms from the main channels, as well as symptoms of the internal organs. Unlike the *Ling Shu*, which lists symptoms for the excess and deficiency conditions of the luo mai, Yang does not list conditions in that way. Yang makes a major shift and variance from the *Ling Shu* in the functions of the luo points. The following is an example of Yang's presentation of the source–luo point combination from the *Zhen Jiu Da Cheng*.

The Twelve Channels Treat Patterns, Using Host–Guest, Source and Luo Points

Lung as the Host, Large Intestine as the Guest

Taiyin has copious qi and scant blood;

qi distension of the heart and chest, feverish palms.

No one can avoid panting and cough,

pain in supraclavicular fossa;

swollen or dry throat, body sweating more and more.

Pain in the medial anterior shoulder and the two breasts;

phlegm binding the diaphragm, qi is lacking,

What points should we seek for disease which is engendered?

Speak with a gentleman about Tai Yuan (Lung 9)

and Pi Lian (Large Intestine 6).[30]

Now let's compare this function to the one found in the *Ling Shu*. The *Ling Shu* states that the Arm Tai Yin collateral treats:

> **Excess:** Heat in the wrist and the palm.
>
> **Deficiency:** Yawning and frequent urination.

The differences in functions are the inclusion of the Hand Tai Yin main channel (lung channel) and some of the lung organ functions. All three are presented in the appendix.

GEORGE SOULIÉ DE MORANT

George Soulié dé Morant was a pioneer in bringing acupuncture from China to France. He made part of the source–luo point method popular in the western community. His book *Chinese Acupuncture* (1972/1994) is considered the first major book on Chinese medicine in France; the book was to spread throughout the western world. The first volume was published in 1939. The entire book eventually comprised three volumes, and was first published in 1957. After the author's passing, his colleague Dr. Thérèse Martiny spent 15 years compiling Morant's notes and condensing decades of clinical experience. The entire body of work was published in 1972.

Morant studied medicine in China. He cites two important Ming dynasty books as the references for his luo point theory and application. The first text is the *Zhen Jiu Da Cheng* (*The Great Compendium of Acupuncture and Moxibustion*) by Yang Jizhou; and the second is the *Yixue Rumen* (*Introduction to Medicine*) by Li Can.

Morant's method

Morant promotes the use of the luo point to treat any condition of the main channels and the internal organs. He varies from the *Zhen Jiu Da Cheng* in that his first treatment approach is to use only the luo point of the deficient channel or organ. For example, if the bladder was excess and the kidneys deficient, he would reinforce the kidneys. He believed that by reinforcing the kidneys the bladder would be reduced, and a balance would occur between both channels. Instead of using the source and luo point combination to obtain the balance, he uses only the luo point.

Yang Jizhou did not present a theory for how the source–luo point worked. Morant proposed that the luo mai have *transverse* channels where qi and blood can be transferred between the Yin–Yang paired luo mai and the main channels, and the internal organs. For example, when reinforcing Liver 5, the liver luo point, the gallbladder channel and organ will be reduced, balancing both channels. In this theory, treating Liver 5 causes a reaction that brings qi and blood into the liver to strengthen it, and also reduces or pulls away an imbalance in the gallbladder, creating a balance between both channels and organs. The balance occurs by way of the transverse luo channel. This application varies from Yang's treatment, which uses both the source and the luo point. It also varies from any luo mai treatment in the *Ling Shu*. Morant uses the luo points to treat conditions that the source points could treat, choosing the luo point instead of the source point.

WHAT ARE THE LUO MAI?

Morant presents interpretations of the entire channel system that differ from classical Chinese medical sources. He calls the luo collaterals the secondary channels. Chapter V of his book is titled "The Fifteen Secondary Vessels." He states:

> These luo or secondary vessels and their points of passage are an important element in the circulation of energy. They are branches that connect the paired channels; i.e, they send the energy from the yin meridian to its coupled yang meridian and from the yang meridian to its coupled yin meridian.[31]

Morant cites the *Yixue Rumen*:

> The jing meridians are the main pathways, and the secondary vessels are the luo... The luo are what run crosswise.[32]

MORANT'S MAIN NOTION AND ASSUMPTIONS

The following is from Morant's *Chinese Acupuncture*.

> The functions of the luo are not explained with complete clarity. Nonetheless, it has been possible to deduce two functions:
>
> 1. To allow the excess energy from a meridian to pass into a paired meridian. This occurs when the normal passage of energy from one meridian to another (the primary channels) is not sufficient to relieve excess. The secondary vessels (luo collaterals) take up this excess energy.
>
>   These luo or secondary vessels and their points of passage are an important element in the circulation of energy. They are branches that connect the paired channels; i.e., they send the energy from the yin meridian to its coupled yang meridian and from the yang meridian to its coupled yin meridian. Any given meridian has a point of excitation or point of passage. When the jing (meridians) are functioning normally, the courses of the secondary vessels are not easily perceived.
>
> 2. They also re-establish the circulation in a meridian. [33]

Morant states that if a meridian is empty and its coupled meridian is full, tonification of the point of passage (luo point) of the empty meridian is enough to replenish it, while at the same time the coupled meridian in excess will become normal.

Morant's luo channel theory includes the following functions.

1. The luo collaterals run crosswise. This crosswise (horizontal) luo channel flow is what connects it to its paired channel, and this crosswise channel can transfer qi and blood between the Yin–Yang

paired channels. This crosswise channel is named by Morant the *transverse* luo channel.

2. When there is excess in one channel and a deficiency in its paired channel, treat the deficient channel with a tonification method. For example, if the lung channel is deficient and the large intestine channel is excess, tonify Lung 7, the luo point. According to Morant, this treatment will tonify the lungs and reduce the excess in the large intestine channel. According to this theory, by tonifying Lung 7 the energetic force will direct qi and blood from its paired channel into the lungs. This movement will tonify the lungs and reduce the excess in the large intestine.

Evaluating Morant's theory

Morant calls the luo mai the secondary vessels. It is common to define the secondary vessels as the muscle channels (sinew channels), luo collaterals, divergent channels and the eight extraordinary channels. Viewing the luo mai as the secondary vessels expands the role of the luo mai as found in the *Ling Shu* and the *Su Wen*. The *Ling Shu* and the *Su Wen* do not describe the luo collaterals as treating the primary channels or the internal organs. Morant does not clearly identify when the luo mai, the primary channels or the internal organs are imbalanced: he does not include a set of symptoms and conditions. He does not describe symptoms when both the lung and the large intestine are imbalanced, as distinct from those when one of the channels is imbalanced; and he does not describe the symptoms of two excesses or two deficiencies.

The *Ling Shu* and the *Jia Yi Jing* (*Classic of Acupuncture and Moxibustion*) present different conditions for the main channels, the internal organs and the luo mai. Morant uses the luo point to treat conditions from all the channel systems and the internal organs. He does not discuss this variance or the reasoning whereby the practitioner would not follow the advice of the *Ling Shu* (Chapter 9): treat points on the two Yin–Yang paired main channels to treat the main channels and the internal organs. He offers no explanation as to why treating one luo point is a more effective method.

The following are the main areas of Morant's theory that require analysis.

1. The *Nei Jing* clearly states that pathogens can be transferred from the luo mai to the primary channels and the internal organs, if they are not treated when they are in the luo mai. *Pathogens* can transfer, but the classics do not say the luo mai can transfer qi and blood to balance the main channels and the internal organs.

2. The *Nei Jing* states that the luo points treat the luo mai and their pathology. It clearly describes the luo mai and the conditions related to them. It does not say they treat the internal organs. The *Ling Shu* clearly indicates that to treat conditions of the main channels and the internal organs, treat the main channel points. There is no mention of using luo points. Chapters 9 and 10 of the *Ling Shu* present a sophisticated pulse method (Renying cunkou pulse method) to diagnose the main channels and how to treat them. In Chapter 10 the luo mai are presented. The presentation in the *Ling Shu* clearly describes the differences between the luo mai and the main channels. One important difference is that the luo mai cannot be detected with the pulse, while the main channels can be detected with the pulse. Morant uses the pulse to measure whether there is an imbalance in the Yin–Yang paired channels and whether the luo points should be treated; he is measuring the main channels and using the luo point to treat them, not the luo mai. The *Ling Shu* is clear that when there is an imbalance in the pulse, it is detecting the main channels and the internal organs, and the treatment is to treat the main channels.

3. The *Nei Jing* does not mention transverse luo mai but gives only one luo mai (collateral) description. There are statements throughout the *Ling Shu* about the luo mai; often a line or a few words are extracted and used to support a theory, but when the entire sentence or chapter is evaluated, the extracted interpretation is questionable. The following is an example of this.

Chapter 17 of the *Ling Shu*, "The Limits of the Channels":

> The main channels make the foundation, while the branches are horizontal and make the luo collaterals. These collaterals divide and make tiny branches, and when they are full with blood, quickly drain the collaterals.

This *Ling Shu* reference states that the branches are horizontal and they are the luo collaterals, which are tiny channels. There is no mention of these horizontal channels connecting to the primary channels and the internal organs. It is clear the *Ling Shu* is saying that the horizontal channels (which Morant calls the transverse luo collaterals) are the tiny luo collaterals, and they should be pricked to bleed to release pathogens; there is no mention or reference that they are used to transfer qi and blood to treat imbalances of the main channels and the internal organs. Pathogens in the luo mai can influence the main channels and the internal organs; applying a luo mai treatment removes the pathogens and the effects they have on the main channels and the internal organs. Attempting to transfer qi and blood may transfer pathogens, which can create a more severe condition.

4. Morant says that one channel must be excess and its Yin–Yang paired channel must be deficient as the requirement for treating the luo point. The method is to reinforce the luo point on the deficient channel. This varies from the method in the *Zhen Jiu Da Cheng*, which is to treat the source point on the problem channel and the luo point on the paired channel. This would make sense, as the source point influences the main channels and the internal organs. Because Yang Jizhou offers no needling technique, we can assume he thought the practitioner would know whether to reinforce or reduce. According to Morant, reinforcing the deficient luo point will result in balance between the two channels; both channels will become balanced. This method varies from Yang's clinical application.

5. Morant is not treating the luo mai and their pathology. In common with Yang Jizhou, this leads to the regular usage of luo points to treat conditions of the internal organs and the main channels.

A question arises: if there is lung qi deficiency, would you treat the luo point/Lung 7, the source point/Lung 9, the front mu point/Lung 1, the back shu point/Bladder 13 or the influential point of qi/Ren 17? Why would Lung 7 be more effective than these other points?

6. The *Ling Shu* says the method to treat the luo mai is prick to bleed the luo points, which releases the pathogen from the body. Morant does not use the prick to bleed method; he needles the luo points.

7. Morant presents a case that includes the heart. He suggests treating the small intestine with the heart, because this is the rule of the paired channels. This is also the guidance of Chapter 9 of the *Ling Shu*. However, this treatment is for the main channels, not the luo collaterals. It seems Morant applies to the luo collaterals a treatment plan designed for the main channels. Chapter 9 also suggests needling the paired main channels with a three-point needling strategy: two needles disperse and one needle reinforces; or two needles reinforce and one needle disperses. Morant appears to apply this method for the main channels to luo mai conditions. Morant suggests reinforcing the luo point on the deficient channel and, if this treatment does not work, then try dispersing the luo point (passage point) on the excess organ. He presents a treatment that differs from both the *Zhen Jiu Da Cheng* and the *Ling Shu*.

A basic question would arise: why would a practitioner use the luo mai and the luo points to transfer qi and blood to another channel system and the internal organs? One possibility is that the creators of this method did not use the luo mai and the other channel systems (muscle, divergent and eight extraordinary channels) in a comprehensive way in clinical practice. Due to not using the entire channel system, they may have sought to treat all conditions with the channels and points they commonly used—which are the main channels and the special points. This approach leads to the expanded use of the luo points beyond treating luo mai conditions.

DR. NGUYEN VAN NGHI AND DR. ALBERT CHAMFRAULT

Dr. Nguyen Van Nghi (NVN) was born in Vietnam and was one of the most important scholars, writers, teachers and practitioners of modern times. Many of his theories and applications are the source for many modern teachers from Europe and the United States. NVN was an allopathic physician. He studied Chinese medicine after practicing western medicine. NVN was to dedicate his life to Chinese medicine.

NVN moved to France and eventually collaborated with French practitioners. A significant collaboration was with Dr. Albert Chamfrault, who carried on the tradition of Morant. Through this collaboration it appears that NVN integrated some of the language Morant used into his own explanation of Chinese medicine. Chamfrault and NVN expand on Morant's theory of transverse luo collaterals and the transfer of qi by using the luo and source points. They promote combining the source and the luo point to transfer qi between the channels. The transfer is through the transverse luo collateral. (As already stated, there is no mention of transverse luo branches in any classic Chinese medical texts.)

A common area of controversy is some practitioners' interpretation of Chapter 63 of the *Su Wen*, "Acupuncturing the Superficial Luo." Chamfrault and NVN reference Chapter 63 to support the transfer theory. The chapter describes how pathogens in the luo mai can be transferred through the body, and presents a special needling method, opposite side needling (mui ci), to treat certain conditions. It describes how pathogens in the luo mai can transfer to the side opposite the origin of the condition. Because of this transfer, contralateral needling is advised. In this specific case, when contralateral needling is applied the treatment is actually at the origin of the condition. Awareness of this transfer of pathogens through the body may have led Chamfrault and NVN to expand Morant's view that the source and luo points can transfer qi and blood throughout the channel system, and according to them, it is the transverse luo mai that is the path that transfers the qi and blood. This view ignores one essential understanding of the luo mai: they are used to remove pathogens from the body with the prick to bleed technique, and if the pathogens are not removed, they can transfer to the main channels and the internal organs and to all the areas in which they flow.

Chapter 63, "Acupuncturing the Superficial Luo," is used to support new ideas in the practice of acupuncture. Some modern teachers reference this chapter as the source of divergent channel theory, not the luo mai. There is one reference to "bie" in the chapter. "Bie" means "diverts" (separates from the main channel). The meaning is the same as "branches." If you read Chapter 63 you will see more than 20 references to the luo and only one for bie. One of the supporting arguments for this new theory is that the pathology listed in Chapter 63 can include conditions in the big joints (articulations), and that the big joints are where the divergent channels flow, whereas the luo mai do not flow there. This theory ignores one main aspect of the luo mai: pathogens can transfer from the luo mai to the main channels and the internal organs, and to all the areas where they flow. Chapter 63 explains this type of transfer through the body. The chapter states:

> When a pathogen invades the body it first enters the skin level. If it lingers and is not treated it will travel into the smaller luo. If the pathogen is not released from the smaller luo it will travel to the main luo mai. If the pathogen is not treated it will flow to the main channels, and then to the five zang organs, and then to the intestines and stomach. The pathogen may now affect everything (all areas of the body).

This passage describes the transfer of pathogens from the luo mai to the main channels, to the internal organs, and potentially they can flow everywhere. In this condition it would be normal for luo pathogens to flow to all the joints, small and large; these are the pathways of the luo mai, the main channels and the divergent channels.

The opening sentences of Chapter 63 include the statement: "I have heard of a technique that applies acupuncturing the 'superficial luo.'" This makes it clear that Chapter 63 is about the luo mai.

The transfer of qi and blood in the way Chamfrault and NVN propose is an entirely new idea in Chinese medicine. The theory is rooted in the *Zhen Jiu Da Cheng*, adapted by Morant, and expanded further by Chamfrault and NVN. Chamfrault and NVN provide their own theory which is not found in any of the earlier Chinese medical classics. NVN differs from Morant in that he suggests always treating the luo and source point combination. He says the transverse channel flows from the luo point to the source point. Also, both Morant and NVN suggest the widest range of conditions can be treated using their methods: any condition of the main channels and the organs. The creation of the transverse luo theory is an attempt to explain how the *Zhen Jiu Da Cheng*'s source–luo point combination functions.

Summary of Dr. Nguyen Van Nghi's teachings

NVN indicates that there are two kinds of collateral within the luo mai. The first are the pathways presented in the *Ling Shu*. He calls these the *longitudinal luo collaterals*. He says there are also pathways from the luo point (which he calls a reunion point, not the point of separation) to the paired Yin–Yang channel. These pathways are labeled the *transverse luo collaterals*. This explanation can be viewed as formulating a theory to support Morant's thesis about the transfer of qi and blood. Unlike Morant, NVN uses the *Zhen Jiu Da Cheng*'s source and luo point combination, with the transfer of qi and blood between those two points by way of the transverse luo pathway. This theory is used to support NVN's source and luo point treatment.

The classics present the theory that the luo mai are located at the superficial layer of the body and are treated with the prick to bleed method to release the pathogen(s). If pathogens are not released, they can transfer to the main channels and the internal organs. The *Ling Shu* meticulously describes the functions and symptoms of the main channels, and distinguishes them from luo mai symptoms. The *Ling Shu* recommends treatment plans that balance the main channels and the internal organs.

Morant says the source of the source–luo point theory is found in the *Zhen Jiu Da Cheng*. He says he found in his clinical practice that treating the luo point alone could effectively balance the paired Yin–Yang channels. In his theory, he is influencing not only the luo mai, but also the primary channels and the internal organs. Morant continues the *Zhen Jiu Da Cheng*'s usage of luo points, and expands upon the conditions found in the *Zhen Jiu Da Cheng*, but this is questionable and not supported with theory and references. Because he does not list the conditions that can be treated with the luo points, he leaves wide open the possible conditions they can treat; he implies that any condition of the main channels and the internal organs can be treated in this way.

NVN expands Morant's theory and says that the transverse luo collaterals are a circuit from the Yin–Yang channels. His theory is that there is a transfer from the luo mai to the primary channels and the internal organs. He concludes that the luo point is the connection to the luo collaterals, and the source point is the connection to the primary channels and the internal organs. Treating the two channels at once transfers pathogens or qi from the two channel systems. This view is not found in the *Ling Shu* or the *Su Wen*. This method requires caution to avoid transferring pathogens to the main channels and the internal organs. A clear explanation is needed of when not to use this method.

SUMMARY

The *Ling Shu* presents the luo mai pathways and the conditions they treat. The *Zhen Jiu Da Cheng* presents a new point combination, the source–luo point combination, which is called the host–guest. The *Zhen Jiu Da Cheng* recommends treating the source point of the problem channel and the luo point for its paired Yin–Yang channel, and says that the combination can treat patterns of the 12 channels. In this method the luo point can assist in treating the main channels and the internal organs.

The *Zhen Jiu Da Cheng* does not contain any reference for source–luo point treatment. (Yang Jizhou typically lists sources.) The book does not recommend a needling technique: whether to reinforce or reduce. And there is no guidance for what the luo point treats and what the source point treats. There is no theory about how this method works, and there is no discussion about how this point combination might be better than treating points on the main channels. In the Ming dynasty needling was the common treatment method, and the prick to bleed method was not common. The shift away from the prick to bleed method seems to have led practitioners to try to needle channels and points to treat pathogens that according to the *Ling Shu* and the *Su Wen* require prick to bleed. Additionally, there was a shift to using one channel system (the main channels) to treat conditions beyond their classic functions.

NVN expands on Morant's theories. He indicates that the luo mai have two branches: the first is the longitudinal branch and the second is the transverse branch. These are terms devised by the French practitioners and NVN. NVN defines their function: he proposes the transverse luo is where a transfer of qi and blood occurs in the luo mai. This is not found in the early Chinese medical classics. The *Ling Shu* clearly says that pathogens can transfer from the luo mai to the main channels and the internal organs (in some cases throughout the entire body). NVN varies from this classic understanding of the luo mai and conveys that the practitioner can transfer qi and blood through the transverse channels. The *Ling Shu* clearly advises practitioners to use the Yin–Yang main channels to transfer qi and blood through their paired channel relationship, in order to treat the main channels and the internal organs. Both Morant and NVN vary from this *Ling Shu* guidance. The *Ling Shu* states that the luo mai can release pathogens in the body, and the method is prick to bleed.

The ancient practitioners presented a comprehensive medicine and channel system; it is clear that they were conveying a highly detailed understanding of the human body and effective ways to treat illness. The purpose of this chapter has been to stimulate an exploration of the Han dynasty classical methods of the luo mai by comparing them to a modern theory and its clinical applications. As practitioners of this ancient healing system, one part of our learning process is to follow the path handed down from the originators of this medicine. As we trace the steps of those profound healers, we develop the knowledge to evaluate current theories and clinical applications. A goal of this process is to reach our full potential as Chinese medical practitioners. Studying the classics is an important means to that end.

Chapter 10

CLINICAL STRATEGIES FOR TREATING EMOTIONS AND SHEN DISTURBANCES

Chinese medicine is holistic medicine. An important aspect of holistic medicine is that there are multiple causes of health conditions and numerous ways to treat them. In Chinese medicine, holistic models of diagnosis and treatment developed. One holistic model is the three treasures: Jing–Qi–Shen. These treasures correspond to the physical, mental (emotional) and spiritual qualities of each person. Practitioners can view every condition through the lens of Jing–Qi–Shen; a goal is then to identify which of the treasures is influenced. Each of the treasures can influence the others, and treatment can include treating one, two or three of the treasures. For example, psycho-emotional conditions can influence the physical body. A person may have anger that causes muscle tension. Another example is a person suffering from chronic, intense fear. The fear influences the kidneys and the bladder, causing frequent and urgent urination. These two examples are situations where emotions influence the physical body. The early Chinese healers understood that each person was an integration of physical, mental and spiritual energies, and they presented numerous ways to treat multi-dimensional people. Effectively treating a wide range of psycho-emotional conditions requires comprehensive use of the acupuncture channel system.

When treating psycho-emotional conditions and the Shen, it is common to treat multiple channel systems. The first analysis is to determine if the condition is acute or chronic. If it is acute, it is common to treat the luo mai. If the condition influences the musculoskeletal system, then including the muscle channels (sinew channels) in the treatment will make the treatment more effective. If the condition influences the internal collateral organs—for example, nausea, vomiting or loss of appetite—adding the main channels to the treatment will make it more effective. Identifying which areas of the body are influenced by the psycho-emotional condition is essential in effective treatments.

THE LUO POINTS

The luo points can be used to treat their corresponding collateral and shen. There are a variety of ways to treat the Yin and Yang luo points. I have found a treatment to be most effective when both are included in it. The classic method is prick to bleed. This method can include using a lancet. Lancets can be challenging for practitioners to use if they are not trained in the method; plum blossoming is a very effective alternative to a lancet. The treatment goal is to remove the pathogen from the body. Needling superficially would be a third option.

There are several ways to use the luo points in a treatment. The following is a list of eight ways to use luo points for treating psycho-emotional conditions.

1. Treat the Yin luo point.
2. Treat the Yang luo point.
3. Treat the Yin and Yang luo points on Yin–Yang paired channels.
4. Combine the Yin luo point on the imbalanced channel with other channels' luo points.
5. Combine the Yang luo point on the imbalanced channel with other channels' luo points.
6. Combine the Yin and Yang luo points on the imbalanced channels with other channels' luo points.
7. Use the luo points with points from other channel systems. In this situation, use the luo point to release the pathogenic factor and qi.
8. Combine window of the sky points with luo points.

EXAMPLES OF APPLYING THE LUO POINTS

1. Treat the Yin luo point

The *Nei Jing* states the Yin organs house the five shen. Imbalances of the shen can be treated with the Yin luo points. They can release the intensities and emotional imbalances of the shen. It is most effective to treat these points bilaterally. You can needle the points according to gender: the right side is Yin and females, and the left is Yang and males.

2. Treat the Yang luo point

Yang organs empty; they release and let go. Yang organs should not be full. The fundamental energetics of Yang organs is to release. To release emotions, treat the Yang luo point of the corresponding organ and shen; this will release the emotionally charged energy. This method is a powerful way to obtain a quick emotional release.

3. Treat the Yin and Yang luo points

In my experience, treating both the Yin and Yang luo points is the most powerful method. My preferred method is to treat the Yin luo on the right side of the body and the Yang luo on the left side of the body. I use two points for most conditions. If there was a severe condition, I would treat both points bilaterally. Ideally, plum blossom both points. An alternative method is to needle the Yin luo point and plum blossom (or lancet) the Yang luo point. Needling the Yin luo point sends a message to the body that the channel, organ and shen are to be treated. Treating the Yang luo paired point releases the pathogen or emotionally charged qi. Prick to bleed is the most powerful method. If needling is performed it should be done superficially with a reducing method. Gua sha can also be applied instead of plum blossoming.

4. Combining a Yin luo point with luo points from other channels

It is common that two or more of the five shen are imbalanced. The cause of an imbalance can follow the five phases cycles: the parent, the same, the child, the grandparent and the grandchild relationships. There can be too much or too little of these relationships, creating an imbalance. When there is more than one shen imbalanced, we can treat them. For example, a common diagnosis is wood overacting on earth. This can be liver qi stagnation, and the liver overacts on the spleen. When emotions are the cause of this dynamic the diagnosis can be a hun and yi disharmony. The treatment can be the luo points on both of these channels.

The Yin luo points on the imbalanced channels can be treated. For example, Liver 5 and Spleen 4 can be treated in a hun and yi disharmony. The two Yang luo points can be treated as well, which are Gallbladder 37 and Stomach 40. Both the Yin and Yang luo points on the channels can be treated: Liver 5, Gallbladder 37, and Spleen 4 and Stomach 40. Ideally, they all are bled with either a lancet, plum blossom or gua sha. There are various ways to sequence the order of insertion of treatment. The first is the order just listed. It would be left then right, or right then left. Another way is to treat the two Yin luo points and then the two Yang luo points. My preference is to treat the Yin luo point on the right side and then the Yang luo point on the left side.

5. Use the luo points with points from other channels

In this method the luo point is an outlet. The practitioner selects a point to be reduced on the imbalanced channel and then treats the luo point to release the pathogen or energy. For instance, a patient has a yi disharmony with obsessive thinking. The patient also has a headache. The treatment is to needle Stomach 8 on either the right or the left side, and then treat Stomach 40 on the same side. The two points are on the same channel and the reducing method on Stomach 8 begins to move the pathogen outward, with treatment of the luo channel releasing it from the body. I have found this to be a very effective treatment. It can be applied to all the channels and the five shen. The point combination of the window of the sky points with luo points is another version of this type of treatment plan.

The Chinese medical classics present a profound understanding of Shen disturbances. An important part of this understanding is how pathogenic factors cause Shen disturbances. An excellent book on this subject is *Shen Disturbance: A Guideline for Psychiatry in Traditional Chinese Medicine*, by Joseph Changqing Yang (2005).

The five shen Chinese medical model provides an effective framework for clinical practice. There are a variety of ways to treat areas, pathogenic factors and vital substances that influence the five shen. The following are the main points I use to treat the five shen:

1. Luo points and the luo mai
2. Back shu points
3. Front mu points
4. Well points
5. Source points
6. Sea points
7. Window of the sky points
8. Psycho-emotional points based on name and channel
9. Divergent channel points
10. Extraordinary channel points.

The luo mai and the luo points can release emotional qi and pathogens that can disturb the five shen and the Shen. Treating the luo mai is a major way to treat pathogens that influence emotions and the five shen.

The *Su Wen* says that the five Yin organs house the five shen. The condition of the Yin organs (and the Yang organs, because they influence their paired channels) directly influences the five shen. Points that can influence the organs can influence the five shen. The front mu and the back shu points, especially the Yin back shu points, can treat the organs. The well points are among the most powerful points that influence the main channels and the internal organs. The sea points also influence the internal organs. These points can be reinforced or reduced to influence the internal organs. Reinforcing and reducing techniques can strengthen or clear the internal organs, providing a healthy environment for the five shen. The methods can also reduce pathogens that are in the organs and the channels. The pathogens can disturb the channels, organs, vital substances and the five shen.

In Chapter 8 of this book I presented a theory for treating the window of the sky points. In my experience, the two most effective treatments using the window of the sky points are the following:

1. Needle the source, the window of the sky point and then the luo point. It is best if you prick to bleed the luo point. You can plum blossom the luo point instead of pricking to bleed. You can also needle the luo point superficially; this method is secondary to the prick to bleed method and plum blossom.

2. Needle the window of the sky point and then prick to bleed or plum blossom the luo points. If you can't prick to bleed or plum blossom the luo point you can needle the luo point superficially.

Chapter 5 of the *Ling Shu*, "Roots and Ends," presents the sequence of the well, source, river, window of the sky and luo points. These points are listed in Table 10.1.

Table 10.1 The roots and ends points with luo points

Channel	**Well** Root (begins) Fingers–toes	**Source** Passage Wrist–ankle	**River** Arrival Arm–leg	**Window of the sky** Neck	**Connecting point** Penetration Mid-leg–mid-arm
Tai Yang	Bladder 67	Bladder 64	Bladder 60	Bladder 10	Bladder 58
Shao Yang	Gallbladder 44	Gallbladder 40	Gallbladder 38	Small Intestine 17	Gallbladder 37
Yang Ming	Stomach 45	Stomach 42	Stomach 41	Stomach 9	Stomach 40
Tai Yang	Small Intestine 1	Small Intestine 4	Small Intestine 5	Small Intestine 16	Small Intestine 7
Shao Yang	San Jiao 1	San Jiao 4	San Jiao 6	San Jiao 16	San Jiao 5
Yang Ming	Large Intestine 1	Large Intestine 4	Large Intestine 5	Large Intestine 18	Large Intestine 6

This sequence includes the window of the sky points listed in Chapter 21 of the *Ling Shu*, "Cold and Hot Diseases," except for Lung 3, Tian Fu. Small Intestine 17 is included in this sequence. Small Intestine 17 is one of the ten points listed in Chapter 5 of the *Ling Shu*.

I have found treating the window of the sky point, the source and the luo point on the imbalanced channel is most effective; Table 10.2 lists these points. Table 10.3 lists the window of the sky and the luo points.

Table 10.2 The source, window of the sky and luo points

Name	Source	Window of the sky point	Luo point
Man's Receptor/ Prognosis	Stomach 42	Stomach 9	Stomach 40
Supporting Chimney	Large Intestine 4	Large Intestine 18	Large Intestine 6
Celestial Window	Small Intestine 4	Small Intestine 16	Small Intestine 7
Celestial Shutters/ Appearance	Small Intestine 4	Small Intestine 17	Small Intestine 7
Celestial Pillar/ Window	San Jiao 4	San Jiao 16	San Jiao 5
Wind Pillar/ Celestial Pillar	Bladder 64	Bladder 10	Bladder 58
Celestial Mansion/ Storehouse	Lung 9	Lung 3	Lung 7
Celestial Pool	Pericardium 7	Pericardium 1	Pericardium 6

Table 10.3 The window of the sky and luo points

Name	Window of the sky point	Luo point
Man's Receptor/ Prognosis	Stomach 9	Stomach 40
Supporting Chimney	Large Intestine 18	Large Intestine 6
Celestial Window	Small Intestine 16	Small Intestine 7
Celestial Shutters/ Appearance	Small Intestine 17	Small Intestine 7
Celestial Pillar/ Window	San Jiao 16	San Jiao 5
Wind Pillar/Celestial Pillar	Bladder 10	Bladder 58
Celestial Mansion/ Storehouse	Lung 3	Lung 7
Celestial Pool	Pericardium 1	Pericardium 6

CLINICAL APPLICATIONS FOR TREATING THE FIVE SHEN

An insight of the early Chinese medical healers was that exogenous and endogenous pathogens are the cause of many illnesses. A treatment plan to remove the pathogens is essential in enabling the body to function properly. Enabling the body to function properly provides the environment to heal and rejuvenate. The luo mai have an important function in clearing pathogens. In my experience they have a powerful effect of releasing emotionally charged energy.

There are a variety of ways to treat the Shen, the five shen and emotional energy. The clinical applications presented are treatment strategies, plans and methods I use in my clinic, as well as methods I teach at Chinese medical schools.

I have organized the treatments based on the model of the five shen. It is a practical and clear way to diagnose and treat. The aim of the clinical cases is to provide examples of how to use luo points and other channel points to treat psycho-emotional conditions. Be flexible in developing treatments for your patients. These treatments are guidelines for you. I hope you will use them as a base to create unique treatments for each patient. Constructing treatments unique for each person is the essence of Chinese medicine.

In my experience prick to bleed or plum blossoming is the most effective method for quick relief from emotional and Shen disturbances. Needling the luo points superficially is an option. If you choose to needle the luo points superficially, I suggest needling the front mu or the back shu points with other points that assist in releasing the pathogens and charged emotional energy. Combining these types of points is more effective than needling only one of them. For example, if a patient is suffering from sadness and grief, first reducing Lung 1 and then superficially needling Lung 7 is very effective. Treating Lung 1 begins releasing the emotional energy to the superficial area, and Lung 7 releases it. Reducing Lung 1 can also draw the emotionally charged energy from the body. The combination of the two points creates a synergy to release. Apply this example to all the channels.

Each of the following cases has a treatment plan that may require one or more treatments. There is no fixed time frame for the effects to occur. Classical Chinese medicine includes monitoring the patient's response to the treatment. When the patient responds in the desired way to the treatment, the timing is right to continue to the next stage of the treatment plan. As practitioners, we should be prepared to adjust our treatment based on what actually occurs with the patient. Following the basic Chinese medical diagnostic principles of looking, listening, feeling and smelling, we adjust and respond to what actually occurs with our patients.

CASE STUDIES

THE HEART SHEN

The heart and small intestine points that can be included with luo points are listed in Table 10.4.

Table 10.4 The heart and small intestine points

Well	Source	Luo	Sea	Back shu	Front mu	Window of the sky	Names
Heart 9	Heart 7	Heart 5	Heart 3	Bladder 15	Ren 14		Heart 4, Path to the Spirit
Small Intestine 1	Small Intestine 4	Small Intestine 7	Small Intestine 8	Bladder 29	Ren 4	Small Intestine 16 Small Intestine 17	

Point functions

The Ren and kidney channel points near the heart have a strong influence on the heart shen and the Shen. Tables 10.5 and 10.6 list and expand on some of the points. Refer to the kidney section for detailed information on the kidney channel points. When selecting points for a treatment, consider these points.

Table 10.5 The Ren and kidney channels: Shen-related points

Channel	1st intercostal space	2nd intercostal space	3rd intercostal space
Ren	Ren 20 Hua Gai Florid Canopy	Ren 19 Zi Gong Purple Palace	Ren 18 Yu Tang Jade Hall
Kidneys	Kidney 26 Yu Zhong Lively Center	Kidney 25 Shen Cang Spirit Storehouse	Kidney 24 Ling Xu Spirit Burial Grounds

Table 10.6 The Ren channel: Shen-related points

Ren 20 Hua Gai Florid Canopy	This point can support a person's heart shen to open and blossom like a flower. When a person's Shen has been suppressed or repressed, a treatment with this point can help their Shen open and be expressed.
Ren 19 Zi Gong Purple Palace	Zi Gong is the palace of the purple star, which is the center of the sky or heaven. In Taoist cosmology, the purple star is the entry to heaven; it connects to heaven. At a micro level, it is the center of a person. The center of a person is the Shen. Zi Gong can assist in attuning or guiding a person's focus (yi) with their Shen.
Ren 18 Yu Tang Jade Hall	Yu Tang is the hall to the Shen. This point can guide a person to their Shen. When a person is on a path of self-realization, this point combined with other points supports them on the path to Shen realization.

Heart shen case study

A 35-year-old female was abandoned as a child and went to live with an aunt. The patient has chronic anger and sadness.

The patient has a constitutional hun and po imbalance. The anger is so strong it creates a separation from the heart shen. This hun condition includes the po and the shen. The patient should practice the healing sounds twice a day. She can practice the liver and lung healing sounds. It is always best to practice all of the six healing sounds together to harmonize the five shen.

The first part of the treatment plan is to release the anger and sadness qi. The second part of the treatment plan is to align the patient to her heart shen.

Treatment 1

1. Right Liver 5, Left Gallbladder 37
2. Right Lung 7, Left Large Intestine 6.

Plum blossom all the points to release the anger and sadness qi.

Treatment 2

1. Needle and reduce Right Liver 14, then plum blossom Right Liver 5. Repeat this for the left side. This treatment clears anger qi from the liver organ. Liver 5 allows an outlet for this anger qi.
2. Plum blossom Left and then Right Small Intestine 7. This treatment clears heart heat and heart shen excess. The small intestine is a Yang channel, which corresponds to the left side; begin the treatment on the left side.

TREATMENT 3

1. Reinforce Right Kidney 6 and then reinforce Left Kidney 6.
2. Reinforce Right and then Left Liver 9.
3. Needle Right and then Left Heart 4. Slide the needle to the middle depth with no stimulation.
4. Needle Du 22. Slide it back towards the back of the head. No stimulation.
5. Needle Ren 17. Slide it downwards towards Ren 12; no stimulation.

Kidney 6 is Shining Sea and is on the Yin Qiao channel; it guides the treatment inward. Liver 9 is Yin wrapper; it wraps the treatment inward. This inward movement at the ankle and the knee has a synergistic effect. Heart 4 is Path to the Dao; this point guides the treatment to the heart shen. Du 22 is Fontanel Meeting; it guides the treatment into the Jing-Shen (the brain). Ren 17 is Chest Center; it is the front mu of the pericardium and connects the Yi (focus) on the Shen. This treatment should be applied after the excess of the liver hun, lung po and heart shen is cleared. This treatment is designed to guide the patient's attention (focus, yi) internally on her Shen, which is a Shen realization treatment.

THE LUNG PO SHEN

The lung and large intestine points that can be included with luo points are listed in Table 10.7.

Lung 3 is the window of the sky point. Lung 3 can be combined with the luo point in a two-point combination. It can also be combined with the source and luo points in a three-point combination. Lung 8 is Channel Ditch. This point can be used to release emotions and experiences that have been buried in the ditch of the lungs, which influences the po shen. Large Intestine 18 is the window of the sky point. It can be combined with the luo point or with the source and luo point.

Table 10.7 The lung and large intestine points

Well	Source	Luo	Sea	Back shu	Front mu	Window of the sky	Names
Lung 11	Lung 9	Lung 7	Lung 5	Bladder 13	Lung 1	Lung 3	Lung 8, Channel Ditch
Large Intestine 1	Large Intestine 4	Large Intestine 6	Large Intestine 11	Bladder 25	Stomach 25	Large Intestine 18	

Lung po case study

A 55-year-old male was in the process of being divorced by his wife. He was very depressed. His normal temperament is happy and positive.

The diagnosis is a lung po imbalance. The treatment plan is to release the depression energy from the lungs and balance the po.

Treatment

1. Reduce Right Lung 3, and then reduce Right Lung 7. Repeat reducing those two points on the left side.
2. Reduce Right Lung 1 and then reduce Right Lung 8. Repeat reducing those two points on the left side.

Lung 3 is the window of the sky point and Lung 7 is the luo point. Reducing both clears the emotional qi related to the lung po. Reducing Lung 1 assists in clearing the emotional qi from the lungs (the channel and the organ). Lung 8 is Channel Ditch and it is the horary point; it assists in clearing the emotional energy from the lungs.

THE KIDNEY ZHI SHEN

The kidney and bladder points that can be included with luo points are listed in Table 10.8. The functions of select kidney points are described in Table 10.9.

Table 10.8 The kidney and bladder points

Well	Source	Luo	Sea	Back shu	Front mu
Kidney 1	Kidney 3	Kidney 4	Kidney 10	Bladder 23	Gallbladder 25
Bladder 67	Bladder 64	Bladder 58	Bladder 40	Bladder 28	Ren 3

Table 10.9 Functions of select kidney points

Name	Function
Kidney 6 Zhao Hai Shining Sea	This point supplements Yin. It can guide the yi and focus inward to the kidneys and the zhi. It can be combined with other points to harmonize the zhi and the shen.
Kidney 16 Huang Shu Vitals Shu	This point harmonizes the kidneys and the heart, the zhi and the shen.
Kidney 23 Shen Feng Spirit Seal	This point can harmonize kidney Yin and heart Yang. The emphasis is on Yin and Yang. When there is an imbalance of both kidney Yin and heart Yang, this point assists in balancing them.
Kidney 24 Ling Xu Spirit Ruins	This point integrates kidney Yin with the heart. The emphasis is on kidney Yin. Ling is the Yin aspect of the Shen.
Kidney 25 Shen Cang Spirit Storehouse	This point assists in transforming heart fire into shen. The emphasis is on the heart shen.
Kidney 26 Yu Zhong Lively Center	This point allows a smooth flow of qi into the chest and through the channel. The emphasis is on lifting the spirits.

Kidney zhi case study

A 58-year-old female is an executive at a large advertising company. She has been in this industry for 30 years. She suffers from a loss of passion and purpose in her life. She is both physically and emotionally fatigued.

The patient has a kidney zhi and heart shen disharmony. She is also deficient in kidney qi.

The treatment includes the following:

1. Harmonize Shao Yin: the kidneys and the heart, the Jing and Shen, and the zhi and shen.

2. Reinforce the kidneys.

Treatment 1

1. Reinforce Kidney 6 and Kidney 16.
2. Reinforce Heart 4.
3. Insert the needle towards the back of the head for Du 20; no stimulation.
4. Insert the needle towards the abdomen for Ren 17; no stimulation.

Kidney 6 and Kidney 16 reinforce the kidneys and the zhi. These two points combined with Heart 4 (Path to the Dao) integrates and connects Shao Yin, which includes the zhi and the heart shen. Du 20 guides the treatment into the brain (Jing–Shen). When Du 20 is combined with Ren 17, it unites Jing–Shen, and the zhi and the shen.

Treatment 2

1. Left Heart 7, Right Small Intestine 3, Right Kidney 3 and then Left Bladder 65. This point combination is the second set of the channels in the Ying Qi cycle (meridian clock): the heart, small intestine, bladder and kidney channels. These points enhance the circulation of qi within these channels and organs, to energize and revitalize them.
2. Ren 4, Gallbladder 25, Ren 17. Ren 4 reinforces the kidneys and the zhi. Gallbladder 25 is the front mu of the kidneys and reinforces the kidneys and the zhi. Ren 17 connects and aligns the zhi and the shen. This point combination reinforces the kidneys and the zhi and willpower. Needling Ren 17 guides the zhi (willpower) to connect to the heart shen.

Treatment 3

Kidney 6, Heart 7 and Ren 20.

Kidney 6 and Heart 7 (Spirit Gate) connect the zhi and the shen. Ren 20 is Florid Canopy; this point can assist in allowing the patient's flower (spirit) to open and bloom. This is a type of Shen realization.

This treatment is about timing. As practitioners, we learn when a patient is ready for this experience: when excesses have been cleared, the channels opened, the Qi is allowed to flow normally and deficiencies are supplemented, the patient is ready for this type of unfolding and self-realization. With experience you will become effective in knowing the right time for this type of treatment.

THE LIVER HUN SHEN

The liver and gallbladder points that can be included with luo points are listed in Table 10.10.

Liver hun case study

A 36-year-old woman works full-time, has two children, is single and is the sole provider for her family. She suffers from fatigue, irritability, frustration, insomnia and temporal headaches.

The patient has liver qi stagnation and a liver hun imbalance. There is also spleen qi deficiency.

Treatment 1

The treatment plan is to move liver qi and clear the liver hun emotional energy.

1. Plum blossom Right Liver 5 and then Left Gallbladder 37. This treatment clears the liver hun emotional energy.

2. Reduce Left Liver 14 and then Left Liver 5. Reduce Right Liver 14, then Right Gallbladder 37. This treatment clears the emotional energy from the liver and gallbladder organs and channels.

Table 10.10 The liver and gallbladder points

Well	Source	Luo	Sea	Back shu	Front mu	Names
Liver 1	Liver 3	Liver 5	Liver 8	Bladder 18	Liver 14	Liver 4, Mound Center, Metal Point; Liver 9, Yin Wrapper
Gallbladder 44	Gallbladder 40	Gallbladder 37	Gallbladder 34	Bladder 19	Gallbladder 24	Gallbladder 13, Root Spirit

Treatment 2

The treatment plan is to promote the smooth flow of liver qi and reinforce the spleen.

1. Reinforce Right San Jiao 3 and Right Liver 3. Repeat this sequence on the left side. This point combination circulates qi throughout the three jiao.
2. Reinforce Left Spleen 6 and then Left Stomach 36. Needle Du 20, inserting it back towards the neck. Reinforce Spleen 6 and then Stomach 36 on the right side and re-stimulate Du 20. This point combination reinforces the spleen and the stomach.

THE SPLEEN YI SHEN

The spleen and stomach points that can be included with luo points are listed in Table 10.11.

Table 10.11 The spleen and stomach points

Well	Source	Luo	Sea	Back shu	Front mu	Window of the sky	Names
Spleen 1	Spleen 3	Spleen 4 Spleen 21	Spleen 9	Bladder 20	Liver 13		Spleen 16, Abdominal Lament
Stomach 45	Stomach 42	Stomach 40 Stomach 18	Stomach 36	Bladder 21	Ren 12	Stomach 9	Stomach 23, Supreme Unity

Spleen yi case study

A 65-year-old male has gas and bloating and is very fatigued. He also has a big appetite throughout the day and evening. He is worried all the time, and that creates stress.

The patient has spleen and stomach qi deficiency, stomach heat and a spleen yi disharmony. The treatment plan is first to clear stomach heat and harmonize the spleen yi, and then reinforce the spleen and stomach.

Treatment 1

1. Plum blossom Right Spleen 4 and then Left Stomach 40.
2. Reduce Stomach 21 and then Stomach 44. Needle first the left side and then the right side.

Plum blossoming Spleen 4 and Stomach 40 treats the luo mai to get relief from the overactive yi (worrying). Reducing Stomach 21 and Stomach 44 clears stomach heat. The two treatments reduce heat in the stomach and clear emotional qi from the overactive yi.

Treatment 2

1. Perform a shallow-level reducing technique on Right Spleen 4 and then Left Stomach 40.
2. Reinforce Spleen 3, Stomach 36 and then Ren 12.
3. Reinforce San Jiao 6.

Shallow needling continues clearing the emotional qi (worrying). Reinforcing Spleen 3, Stomach 36 and Ren 12, the source, sea and front mu points of the spleen and the stomach, reinforces the stomach and the spleen. Reinforcing San Jiao 6 assists in distributing the treatment throughout the whole body (three jiao).

Table 10.12 lists the luo points for the Yin–Yang collaterals.

Table 10.12 Luo points for the Yin–Yang collaterals

Channel	Yin luo point	Yang luo point
Lung, Large Intestine	Lung 7	Large Intestine 6
Spleen, Stomach	Spleen 4	Stomach 40
Heart, Small Intestine	Heart 5	Small Intestine 7
Kidney, Bladder	Kidney 4	Bladder 58
Pericardium, San Jiao	Pericardium 6	San Jiao 5
Liver, Gallbladder	Liver 5	Gallbladder 37
Spleen	Spleen 21	
Ren	Ren 15	
Du	Du 1	

SUMMARY

The acupuncture channel system includes the muscle (sinew) channels, luo collaterals, main channels, divergent channels and the eight extraordinary channels. Applying all of these channels in clinical practice follows the tradition of the *Ling Shu* and the *Su Wen*. In my experience, the best clinical results occur when using all the channels. The cases presented above introduce ways to use the luo points and a variety of other points to treat emotions and the Shen. The cases should be used as guides for practitioners to formulate their own treatments for each patient. Including the other channel systems is often essential in treatment. Please refer to my other books to learn how to include the other channels in the practice of acupuncture.

CHAPTER 11

THE HEALING SOUNDS

Natural healing practices are a significant contribution from Chinese culture. One of the oldest and most important natural healing practices is qi gong (dao yin). A unique aspect of qi gong is that it can be incorporated into daily life without having to visit a practitioner; and it can be practiced in the comfort of a home, office, backyard or park. Daily practice influences health, vitality and well-being.

Qi gong is a general term that includes a wide range of postures, movements, breath and sound practice. Medical qi gong is targeted to treat specific conditions. This natural healing system includes the principles of Chinese medicine. The healing sounds are a medical qi gong.

The ancient Chinese perceived that humanity and nature are inseparable. From observing life, they developed models that expressed the relationships they saw in it. The models include Yin–Yang, Tai Chi and the five phases. All of life can be viewed in these three flows or patterns. One of the most insightful discoveries of the ancient Chinese was that these models are "systems of correspondences" (relationships between two or more things). The ability to perceive and predict how one correspondence can influence others is the essence of Chinese medicine. Medical qi gong uses this model as a guide to influence correspondences within the body to obtain health and vitality. The healing sounds qi gong presented in this chapter includes important correspondences of the internal organs and the five shen.

Chapter 5 of the *Su Wen*, "The Manifestation of Yin and Yang from the Macrocosm to the Microcosm," introduces the five shen. The five shen can be viewed as five aspects of a person. They are stored or housed in the Yin organs, and each of the five shen corresponds with one of the five phases (five elements):

- the hun is housed in the liver, which is wood
- the shen is housed in the heart, which is fire
- the yi is housed in the spleen, which is earth
- the po is housed in the lungs, which is metal
- the zhi is housed in the kidneys, which is water.

Systems of correspondences include the relationship between organs, shen and emotions. This model includes the ability to influence one correspondence by influencing a distal or related correspondence. For instance, if the po shen is imbalanced and a person is suffering from sadness, treating the lungs can influence this condition with the practice of acupuncture, by selecting the Hand Tai Yin luo mai (the lung collateral) or other channels that have a direct relationship to the lungs for treatment. For instance, the large intestine channel is the *Yin–Yang* pair of the lungs; the spleen is the *Tai Yin* pair of the lungs, and it is the earth, the parent element of metal. The bladder is the *opposite* pair of the lungs in the Ying Qi cycle (meridian clock), and they share part of the same six-channel name: *Tai* Yang and *Tai* Yin. Each of these channels corresponds to the lungs, based on classical Chinese medical principles, and can be treated to influence the lungs and the po shen.

Emotions are qi, and the healing sounds have a powerful influence on qi and emotions. When emotions are imbalanced, they can alter the way qi flows. Emotions not only influence their own organ's qi flow, they can alter the qi of related organs in their five phases and Chinese medical relationships. For instance, if a person suffers from anger, the liver can overact on earth and cause the spleen to suffer from worry, its corresponding emotion. When the liver overacts on the spleen, worry can cause qi to be stagnant and not flow upward, preventing the development of qi and blood in the lungs and the heart. Understanding that emotions are qi allows the practitioner to use numerous methods (including the healing sounds) to balance qi and emotions.

Each of the five phases has a variety of correspondences. Some of the major correspondences are colors, emotions, organs, sensory organs, shen, sounds and shapes. Table 11.1 contains this information.

Table 11.1 The five phases correspondences

	Wood	Fire	Earth	Metal	Water
Color	Green	Red	Yellow	White	Blue-green Black
Direction	East	South	Center	West	North
Season	Spring	Summer	Indian summer	Fall	Winter
Yin organs	Liver	Heart	Spleen	Lungs	Kidneys
Yang organs	Gallbladder	Small Intestine	Stomach	Large Intestine	Bladder
Sense organs	Eyes	Tongue	Mouth	Nose	Ears
Emotions	Kindness Anger Irritability Frustration	Joy Love Hastiness Impatience Arrogance	Openness, Receptiveness Pensiveness Worry Lamenting	Courage Sadness Loneliness	Gentleness Fear
Spirit	Hun	Shen	Yi	Po	Zhi
Sounds	Shhhh	Hawww	Hoooo	Ssssss	Chuiii (the sound of a wave)
Shape	Rod	Triangle	Rectangle	Sphere	Cascading downward

Medical qi gong uses one or more of the five phases correspondences. The correspondences are included in qi gong to stimulate and influence areas of the body, mind and spirit. One of the oldest and most popular medical qi gong practices is the six healing sounds. The healing sounds are an ancient practice. Tao Hongjing (451–536 AD), is one of the most famous Chinese medical doctors, qi gong and nei gong practitioners, herbalists and San Qing Taoists in Chinese history. He promoted the healing sounds as a medical qi gong practice. Most qi gong forms have many variations; the healing sounds also have numerous versions. All traditions have a sound, and some include postures or shapes that reflect the five phases. There are forms that also include a posture, color and emotions. The healing sounds that contain all of those five phases correspondences are a powerful medical qi gong and an effective emotional transformational medical qi gong.

THE BASICS OF MEDICAL QI GONG

The basic goal of the healing sounds is to influence an organ, its channel and its correspondences by applying the three adjustments of medical qi gong: posture, breath and intention. From a traditional Chinese medical viewpoint, medical qi gong can clear heat or wind and break through qi and blood stagnation. From a psycho-emotional viewpoint, the healing sounds can release unfavorable emotions and allow reconnecting to the natural virtues. From a spiritual viewpoint, the healing sounds attune to the five shen. Attuning to the five shen or the five aspects of consciousness allows a person to unite their yi (their attention) with their qi and body as one integrated whole, allowing the natural expression of harmony and balance. From a shamanic viewpoint, the Wu (healers) of ancient China used qi gong to unite with the spirits of heaven, integrating heaven and earth.

Medical qi gong should contain the three adjustments: posture, breath and intention. The following outlines the basic practice for the healing sounds.

1. Begin the healing sounds by taking a long, gentle, deep breath from the lower dan tian (the lower abdomen).

2. As you inhale, move your arms and body into the proper position and then make the sound while exhaling.

3. Exhaling should be slow, gentle and as long as possible. Keep the body relaxed when doing this qi gong. The eyes are open during exhaling.

4. When you finish exhaling, place your hands over the organ to which the sound corresponds; the palms should face the body. The eyes are closed. You can also place your hands at your knees (see the pictures for each sound.)

5. Move the tip of your tongue to your palate and behind your teeth; this enhances the natural flow and connection of qi in the Du and Ren channels, two of the eight extraordinary channels that flow up the back and down the front of the body.

6. Smile, and place your mind's attention in the organs to which the healing sounds are related; this guides qi into the organs, energizing and rejuvenating them. Additionally, the well, spring and stream points (three of the five transporting acupuncture points) are on the hands, and they are among the most energetically powerful points on the body. Placing the hands over an organ transfers qi to the organ to energize and rejuvenate it.

7. Keep your mind's attention (yi) in the organ as you inhale and exhale. Inhaling guides qi into the organ, and exhaling with your yi in the organ keeps it there, reinforcing and energizing it.

8. Exhaling is the Yang stage; it releases excesses and stagnations and is a reducing method. The eyes are open during the Yang stage, the exhale.

9. The rest, or Yin, stage of the practice is a reinforcing method. The eyes are closed during the Yin stage when there is normal breathing with the hands covering the organ.

THE HEALING SOUNDS PRACTICE

There are two major aspects to the healing sounds practice. The first is to release unfavorable emotions and excesses (including gas, heat, fire, cold, wind, qi and blood stagnations). The second aspect is to allow the natural virtue of the organ and shen to manifest. Releasing unfavorable emotion(s) and excess creates space for the natural virtues to be felt. With continual practice these qualities will enter and permeate the body, nourishing it with natural and favorable virtues. This process allows us to manage our emotional condition, as well as providing the opportunity to take action to change and transform our life.

MEDICAL ASPECTS OF RESPIRATION

Exhaling is the reducing method. It releases unfavorable emotions. It can also release pathogenic factors, for instance wind, heat, fire, damp, phlegm and cold. The releasing or clearing process can assist in creating the smooth flow of qi in the channels and the organs. Exhaling also cools the body.

THE REST PERIOD

The rest period is the reinforcing method. When we place our hands over an organ, qi flows there. The qi nourishes and reinforces the organ. This is a rejuvenation practice.

MEDICAL PRESCRIPTION

When prescribing the healing sounds for medical purposes, a medical prescription should be recommended. This prescription can be two times a day or more, and a particular organ sound can be done 9, 18, 36 or 72 times. To reduce or sedate, make the sound loud. To reinforce, make the sound sub-vocally. As a maintenance practice, make a very low sound.

HOW TO PRACTICE THE HEALING SOUNDS

The lungs and large intestine healing sound

The lungs and large intestine are the metal phase and correspond to the po shen. The color is white, gold and silver. The sound is a hissing sound: "*sssss*." The lungs' and large intestine's unfavorable emotions are sadness, depression, grief and sorrow. Imbalances of the po include feelings of isolation and the inability to forgive. The favorable virtue is courage. The shape is sphere and round; therefore, we take a sphere or round-shaped position in this qi gong. All of these correspondences are included in this medical qi gong practice.

The three adjustments for the lung and large intestine healing sound:

- *Posture:* A sphere or round shape. Notice that the arms in this posture are in a sphere or round shape; see Figure 11.1.
- *Intention:* During the exhale, release the unfavorable emotions, and in the rest stage focus on the favorable ones.
- *Breath:* A long inhale to begin, and a long exhale when making the sound. In the rest stage focus your attention/yi is in the lungs and the large intestine, and breathe naturally.

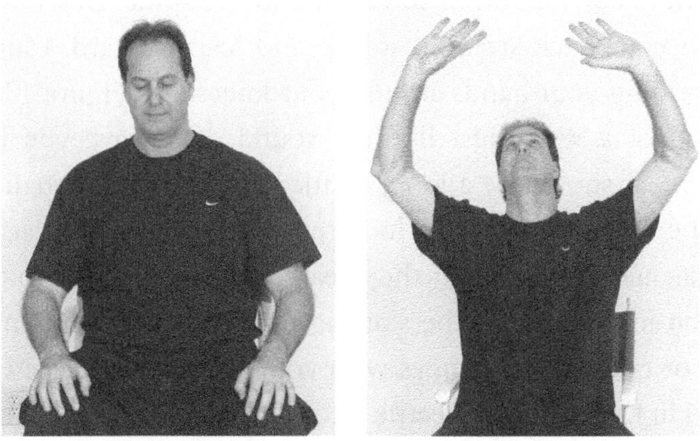

Figure 11.1 The lung and large intestine healing sound

It is traditional to repeat the sound three times. During each season repeat the sound for the season six times. For example, during the fall perform the lung and large intestine sound six times.

The kidney and bladder healing sound

The kidney and bladder correspond to the zhi shen, and to fear and paranoia as well as gentleness. During the exhale release fear, and during the rest period allow gentleness to manifest. The zhi reflects our willpower, and the will to live the type of life we desire. It includes the will to seek and understand our true nature (Shen realization). The kidneys acupuncture channel has an internal pathway that flows to the heart; this is the kidney zhi seeking the heart shen.

The basic nature of water is to be fluid and adaptive, to be able to adjust to any situation. When a person is frozen in life, they become locked and rigid. If the zhi is frozen, fear can manifest; it includes the fear of being trapped and limited. It's a fear that prevents one from changing, from attempting and accomplishing the things that comprise their most innate purpose in life: to live from the heart shen. The kidneys and bladder healing sound can release fear and the coldness that can manifest from being frozen in life.

The kidneys correspond to the back and the spine. Begin by sitting in a chair with your back straight, inhale and lean forward, rounding your back and clasping your hands around your knees (see Figure 11.2). Exhale to the sound of a wave, just like the sound of a wave you hear at the beach: "*chuiii.*" It should be a long, gentle exhale. While exhaling you can just make the wave sound, or include repeating the word "fear," to release any fear that may exist. When the breath has been fully exhaled, slowly inhale as you move back to the starting position. Sit with your hands on your knees or cover your kidneys with your hands, and place your mind's attention/yi in the kidneys. Breathe into the kidneys and exhale into them, keep your yi fixed in the kidneys and repeat the word "gentleness." If you prefer, you can visualize the color blue-green in and around the kidneys.

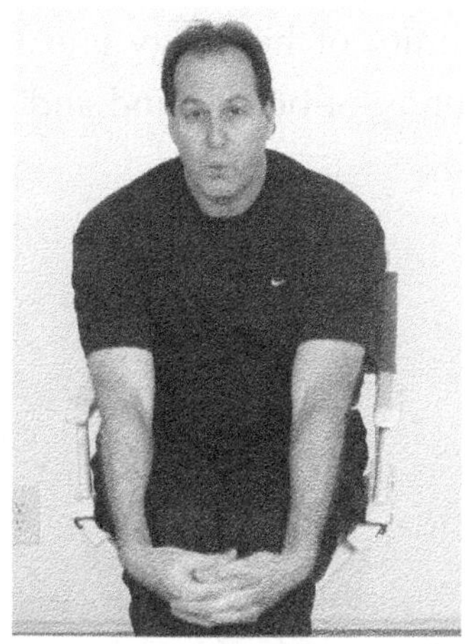

Figure 11.2 The kidneys and bladder healing sound

The exhale releases the negative emotions of the kidneys and the zhi, as well as heat, gas, cold and other pathogenic factors in the channel and the organ. The rest period is the reinforcing stage and strengthens the kidneys. The shape of water is cascading. In this qi gong we move downward and forward—a cascade-like movement. The rounding of the back stimulates the kidneys. This kidneys and bladder healing sound practice combines the sound, emotions, color and the shape of water.

The liver and gallbladder healing sound

The liver and gallbladder correspond to the hun. An imbalanced hun can be expressed as anger, irritability, frustration and a lack of direction. The hun also represents the aspect of our life that allows us to perceive the collective nature of all of humanity and nature. It perceives the unity and the inseparable nature of our life. Wood corresponds to the liver, and when it is imbalanced its energy can rise, float upward and float away. From a psychological viewpoint this can mean a person tries to leave their everyday life, escape or lift up and away from it. This can include denying their physical body. Or it can mean not wanting to interact with people. This leaving can be justified by attempting to be spiritual, being above the physical. Leaving this world is a rejection of the inseparable nature of life, the intrinsic nature of the hun. Its imbalance includes not maintaining its essential quality: the unity of humanity and life. This essential nature includes living from the unity of body, mind and spirit.

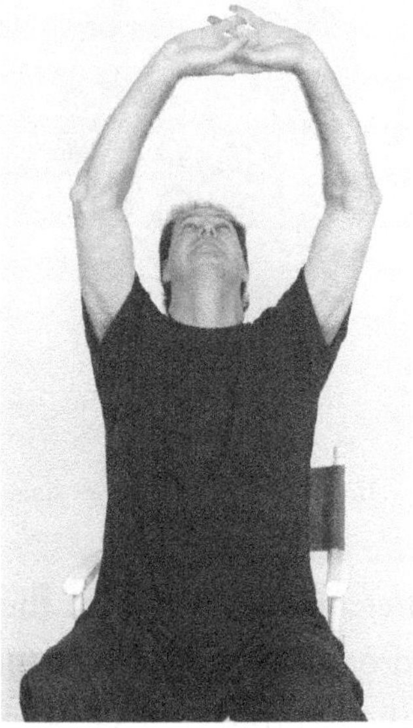

Figure 11.3 The liver and gallbladder healing sound

The liver and gallbladder healing sound is "*shhhh.*" The breathing method for the healing sounds is a long inhale from the lower dan tian, and a long exhale when making the sound. The eyes should be open during the inhalation and the exhalation. Wood is rod-shaped and extends upward. During the sound we assume a rod shape and extend upward. Begin with your hands on your knees, inhale slowly and deeply, and lift your hands up in front of your body, clasp your fingers and extend your hands above your head (see Figure 11.3). Exhale to the "*shhhh*" sound (like you "*shhhh*" a child to be quiet). It should be a long, gentle exhale. You can just make the sound, or you can repeat the emotion for the liver if the emotion is imbalanced, which can be anger, irritability or frustration. If there is an intensity of the emotion(s), make the sound loud. If the healing sounds are practiced as a daily wellness qi gong, make the sound softly.

The rest period is as important as making the sound. When the sound is completed, lower your hands alongside your body and bring your hands near your knees (you can also place your hands over the liver), close your eyes, place your tongue on the palate behind your teeth, and focus your yi/attention in your liver. Close your eyes (always close your eyes in the rest stage) and smile into your liver. If you prefer, repeat the word "kindness" as you smile into the liver. Exhaling and making the sound is the reducing (releasing) stage. The reinforcing stage is when you smile into the organ.

The heart and small intestine healing sound

The heart and small intestine correspond to the heart shen. The color of the heart is red, its shape is a triangle, the direction is south, the planet is Mars, the taste is bitter and the element is fire. The sound is "*hawww.*"

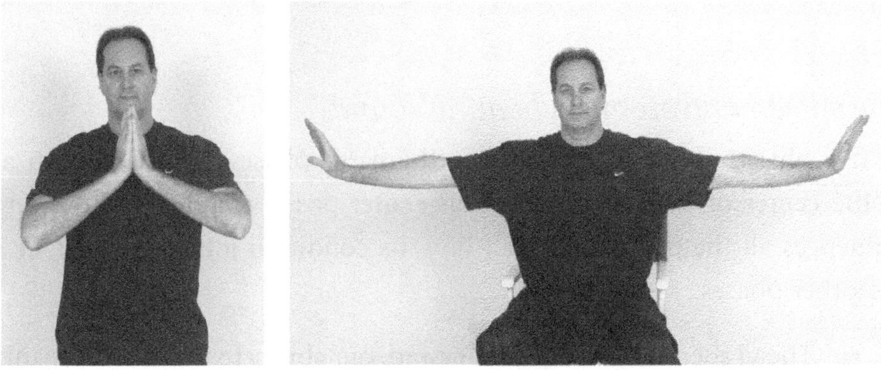

Figure 11.4 The heart and small intestine healing sound

The inhale

The heart and small intestine healing sound has a strong influence on emotions and the Shen. It is essential to clear heat from the heart and any unfavorable qi and emotions from influencing it. The heart and small intestine healing sound is a practical and effective way to harmonize the heart and allow the virtues of joy and love to be naturally expressed in daily life.

Take a long, slow, gentle inhale from your lower dan tian, which includes your lower belly. As you inhale, bring your hands up in a big circle from the sides of the body into a pray posture in front of your body (see Figure 11.4).

The exhale

Perform a long, slow exhale, making the "*hawww*" sound. Extend your arms out to the side of the body and repeat one or more of the following words: "hastiness," "impatience," "arrogance," "cruelty" or "hatred." Release any of these emotions that exist. You can also just make the sound. Stay relaxed while inhaling and exhaling. Do not create any tension in your body during this qi gong. When you have finished exhaling, cover your heart with your hands. Place your intention in your heart and smile. If you prefer, repeat "joy" and "love" silently to yourself as you smile into your heart. Continue smiling to the heart and small intestine for a few minutes until you feel joy and love.

The spleen and stomach healing sound

In five phases and five shen theory, the earth phase and the yi shen are in the center of the five phases. This center position indicates how earth influences all the five phases, and how its condition influences all four of the other phases.

- The yi shen is our conceptual mind, our ability to think and organize thoughts.
- The spleen yi relates to the mouth.
- The kidney zhi is our will and hearing.
- The liver hun represents the ethereal and our ability to understand the collective nature of our life and seeing (eyesight).
- The heart shen represents our essential nature, our purpose, and relates to the tongue and speech.
- The lung po represents the corporeal and the physical body, the nose, breathing and smell.

In the same way as the spleen and stomach are the origin of postnatal essences (they transform and transport food and drink throughout the body), the yi digests, transforms and processes all experiences in our life. All food and drink must go through the mouth; all processing of experiences goes through the yi. The yi transfers these experiences to the other four shen and their corresponding sensory organs. Figure 11.5 illustrates the five shen and the sensory organs. The healing sounds are a way to change the conditioning and patterns formed by the yi.

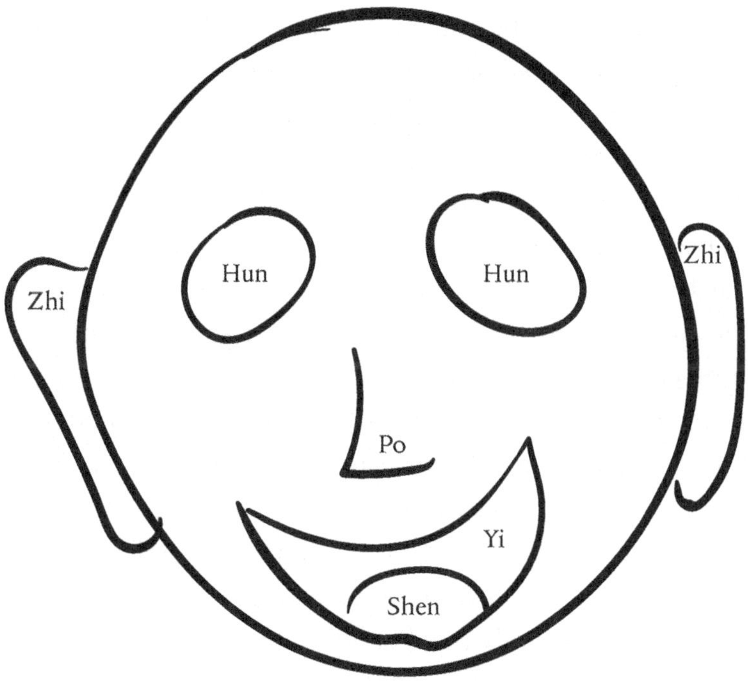

Figure 11.5 The five shen and the sensory organs

The earth is a transforming phase; it receives and processes. The yi is the aspect of our mind that relates to concepts, ideas, thoughts and opinions. The yi takes in experiences and organizes them. The yi makes sense of life experiences, which include feelings and emotions. It is involved in forming the ego. The maturity of the yi contributes to how experiences and emotions are processed. For example, if a person is prejudiced toward a race or ethnic group, this prejudice is part of their thinking and concepts in relation to the group. The person processes this prejudice into the earth yi, which then influences the other shen. How we see (hun), hear (zhi), smell (po) and speak (shen) is influenced by the yi's condition.

A fundamental aspect of the spleen's function is to hold blood in the blood vessels, and assist in circulating blood. On a psychological and emotional level, the yi holds thoughts and feelings inside the body and distributes them throughout the body. If our yi is clear and balanced and is mindful of the innate natural virtues of the five shen, those feelings and virtues are circulated throughout the body. The favorable qualities of the spleen/yi are openness, fairness and receptiveness, including being open to new experiences and the spontaneity of life. The unfavorable qualities include worry, pensiveness, obsessiveness and living in the past—living in past experiences and past conditioned responses to life.

The spleen and stomach healing sound is "*hoooo*" (pronounced like "go"). Begin by sitting in a chair. Your back should be straight and your body relaxed. Open your eyes and slowly inhale, and in a circular movement bring your hands out to the sides of your body, and then gently up to the spleen and stomach area. Place your fingers on your abdomen. Time your inhale to be complete as your hands touch your abdomen. As you exhale, gently move your body a little forward and tuck in your middle abdomen very gently. Make the "*hoooo*" sound as you exhale. You can just make the sound. You can also name and exhale the unfavorable emotion(s), if they exist. After exhaling, gently move back to the beginning position. Place your hands over your abdomen or on your thighs, smile into the abdomen and breathe softly and gently (see Figure 11.6). Keep your intention (focus) in the stomach, spleen and the abdomen. Exhaling is the releasing stage. It releases heat, gas and the unfavorable emotions. The rest stage is the reinforcing stage; it tonifies the spleen and allows the natural virtue of the organ/yi to unfold.

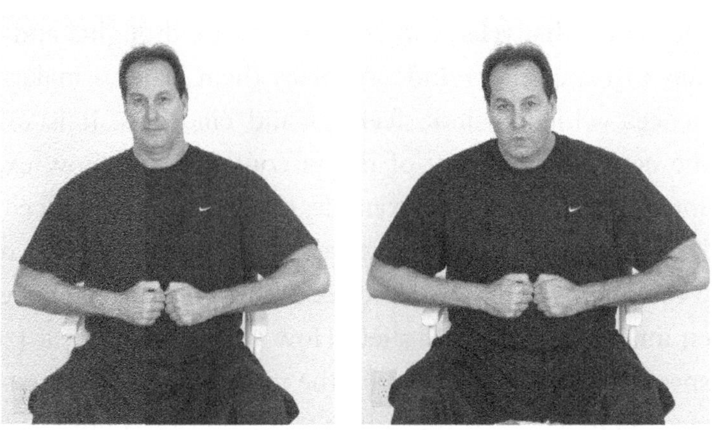

Figure 11.6 The spleen and stomach healing sound

The san jiao healing sound

The san jiao is the last of the six healing sounds. The san jiao is not an organ; it can be translated as the "triple warmer" or "triple burner." The three jiao comprise the lower, middle and the upper areas of the body. The san jiao ranges from the feet to the head. From a qi gong viewpoint, it includes the functioning of the entire body and the circulation of qi throughout the body. One of its major functions is to maintain a balanced temperature in the body. In qi gong it is important to bring heat in the upper areas of the body down to the cooler, lower area of the body, and the coolness of the lower body to the heat in the upper body. When qi is circulating within the body, the heat and the coolness mix to create balanced warmth, promoting health and vitality. In Chinese medicine, the san jiao is involved in two other major functions of the body. The first function is to distribute source qi throughout the entire body. The san jiao also assists in the proper function of water metabolism and fluids throughout the body.

The san jiao influences the entire body. The san jiao healing sound assists in circulating qi through all three jiao, and helps keep a balanced temperature in the body; these two functions are essential for health and vitality.

The san jiao healing sound begins in the sitting position. As you inhale, raise your hands out to the sides of your body and extend them fully up above your head, with the palms facing upward. After a full inhale your hands should be extended above your head. As you exhale, make the "*heeee*" sound (like "tree"). The hands and palms turn inward as you exhale, moving down the front of your body, from above your head and as far as you can down towards your feet. Time your exhale and your arm movement to be completed simultaneously, as your palms move toward the ground. After exhaling, keep your hands at your knees and breathe naturally (see Figure 11.7). Practice the san jiao healing sound three times or more.

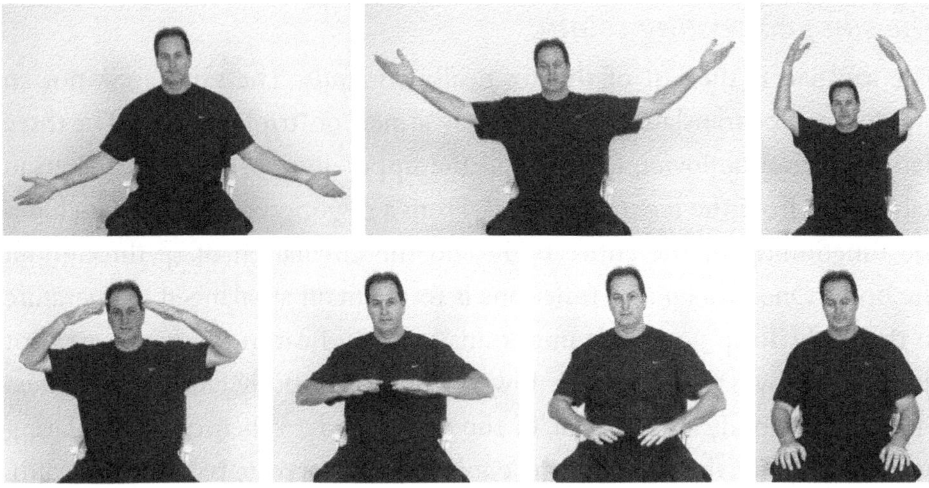

Figure 11.7 The san jiao healing sound

SUMMARY

The healing sounds are a safe, natural way to transform unfavorable emotions, release heat and cool the body. They also tonify the internal organs and allow the natural virtues to unfold. In the Chinese and Taoist model of the three treasures—Jing (Physical), Qi (Energy) and Shen (Spirit)—an individual can be focused more in just one of these aspects of life. If one is stuck in Jing or the physical aspect of life, the physical becomes a predominant focus. The healing sounds can help one to realize that they are not fundamentally their physical body and their emotions. The healing sounds begin a process of becoming more aware of the Qi and Shen aspects of life. As these two aspects of life become the focus of the yi (mindfulness), a balance is achieved among the three treasures. This balance is the foundation of health, happiness and vitality.

Medical qi gong provides an opportunity for people to practice a self-healing method daily in the comfort of their living spaces. The healing sounds can be practiced alone or along with acupuncture and herbal treatments. The combination creates a powerful healing synergy. The healing sounds are a gift from the insights of the early Chinese healers.

APPENDIX

In the Ming dynasty, Yang Jizhou presents new information about the luo points and the conditions they treat. He also presents a new point combination that includes the luo and the source point. In an effort to identify the shift in how the luo collaterals and the luo points are used, I am presenting information about the luo collaterals and the main channels, mainly from the *Ling Shu*[34] among other sources, and then the symptoms and conditions from the *Zhen Jiu Da Cheng*.[35] It can be seen that the *Zhen Jiu Da Cheng* includes conditions from the main channels and the internal organs. Yang does not present excess and deficiency conditions. This expansion of the functions of the luo points is the basis for using them to treat a much wider set of conditions than that found in the *Ling Shu*.

THE LUO COLLATERALS, THE MAIN CHANNELS AND SYMPTOMS AND CONDITIONS

The Hand Tai Yin

- the lungs

THE LUO COLLATERAL

Excess: Heat in the wrist and palm.

Deficiency: Yawning and frequent urination.

The main channel

Conditions include coughing, rebellious qi, panting and thirst, an anxious heart, a congested chest, pain and spasms in the shoulder bone and the medial anterior surface of the upper arm, and heat in the center of the palm.

When the qi is full and there is excess, it results in the shoulder and back being painful from wind and cold. There will be sweating from the attacking wind. Urination is frequent but scanty.

When qi is empty, it results in the shoulder and back being painful from cold. Sparse qi is in accord with an insufficiency of breathing. There will be a change in the color of urine.

Symptoms and conditions from the Da Cheng

Copious qi, scant blood, qi distension of the heart and chest, feverish palms, panting and cough, pain in the supraclavicular fossa, swollen or dry throat, body sweating more and more. Pain in the medial anterior shoulder and the two breasts; phlegm binding the diaphragm, qi is lacking.

The Hand Yang Ming

- the large intestine

The luo collateral

Excess: Toothache, deafness.

Deficiency: Teeth sensitive to cold, bi conditions.

The main channel

There are toothaches and swelling of the neck. This channel transports the body fluids, and may be the source of diseases where the symptoms are yellow eyes, a dry mouth, a runny nose, nosebleed, sore throat, pain in the anterior part of the shoulder or upper arm, and pain and nonfunctioning of the thumb and index finger.

When the qi is in excess, the areas the channel passes through are hot and swollen.

When the qi is empty, the result is cold, chills and poor circulation.

Symptoms and conditions from the Da Cheng

Facial pain, toothache, swollen cheeks. Engendered disease: yellow eyes, the mouth is also dry, runny nose with clear snivel as well as blood gushing, throat impediment (bi), pain in the anterior shoulder, the index finger can be part of the whole (pattern).

The Foot Yang Ming

- the stomach

The luo collateral

Excess: Counterflow qi in the channel, throat bi and sudden loss of voice.

Deficiency: Atony of the feet and a withering of the shins.

The main channel

Diseases include shaking from cold, as if one is sprinkled with water, frequent groaning, frequent yawning, and the forehead is black. A disease state causes the person to feel sick from fire, and to be timid and fearful when hearing tones are resonant to wood. While the heart desires motion, one stays alone behind blocked doors and closed shutters. In extremes, it results in the desire to ascend heights and sing and cast off one's clothes while walking outside. There are noises in the abdomen, and swelling caused by a deficiency around the shinbone. This channel controls the blood and the diseases which arise from it: madness, fevers, warm diseases, debauchery, abnormal sweating, bleeding from the nose, a dry mouth, canker of the lips, swelling of the neck, numbness in the throat, water retention in the abdomen, and swelling and pain in the knee and kneecap.

There is also pain along the shoulder and breast, qi rushing, pain in the abdomen, the thighs, the front of the thigh, the lateral side of the leg bone, the upper part of the foot and ankle, and the middle toe does not function.

When the qi is in excess, it results in the front of the body being hot. So when there is an excess of qi in the stomach, it results in a melting of grains, frequent hunger and yellow-colored urine.

When the qi is insufficient, it causes the front of the body to shiver with cold. When the middle of the stomach is cold, it results in swelling and fullness.

Symptoms and conditions from the Da Cheng

Abdominal fullness, heart oppression, reflection and sorrow; aversion to people, aversions to fire, aversion to light. When the ear hears sounds stirring, there is apprehension in the heart; nosebleeds, deviated lips and malaria also damages, casting off clothes and running around, heat in the body; copious phlegm, foot pain and sores, qi (gu), chest and leg pain that is difficult to stop.

The Foot Tai Yin

- the spleen

The luo collateral

Excess: Cholera, stabbing pain in the intestines.

Deficiency: Drum-like distension of the abdomen.

The main channel

The root of the tongue is rigid, there can be vomiting after eating, and there is pain in the ducts of the stomach, swelling of the abdomen, frequent regurgitation, a gaseous discharge after a bowel movement, and body heaviness. The channel controls the spleen and gives rise to disease where the root of the tongue is painful, the body is unable to move or swing, and food does not descend. There is anxiety in the heart, acute pain below the heart, watery stools, blocked water, yellow jaundice, an inability to lie down, rigidity in standing, swelling and deficiency of the interior of the thighs and knees, and the big toes do not function.

Symptoms and conditions from the Da Cheng

Stiff root of the tongue; vomiting, stomach reflux, diseases of the abdominal viscera, Yin qi surges upward, with belching that is difficult to heal; the body is heavy, the spleen shakes, the affairs of the heart are frenetic, malaria is engendered, shivering, and at the same time emaciation; bound-up stool, yellow jaundice, the hands grasp a cane. The inside of the thighs and knees is swollen, with reversal (cold) and pain.

The Hand Shao Yin

- the heart

The luo collateral

Excess: Fullness and pressure in the chest and diaphragm.

Deficiency: Loss of speech.

The main channel

There is a dry throat and the heart is painful. There is a deficiency of the upper arm. There can be yellow eyes, the ribs hurt, and the medial posterior surface of the upper arm is cold and painful. The center of the palm is hot and painful.

Symptoms and conditions from the Da Cheng

Heart pain and dry throat; thirst and desire to eat, these are arm reversal, engendered disease: yellow eyes, the mouth is also dry; rib-side and arm pain, feverish palms; if the patient desires treatment, do not seek after error; fright palpitations, vomiting blood and fearful throbbing.

The Hand Tai Yang

- the small intestine

The luo collateral

Excess: Loosening of the joints and atony of the sinews in the elbow area.

Deficiency: Small swellings.

The main channel

There can be a sore throat, the chin and jaws are swollen, the neck is stiff and immobile, the shoulder feels as if it is pulled apart, and the upper part of the arm feels as if it is broken. There may be deafness, yellow eyes, swollen cheeks, and pain in the neck, jaws, shoulder, upper arm, elbow and the lateral posterior side of the arm.

Symptoms and conditions from the Da Cheng

Swollen cheeks, shoulder pain, the sides of the two arms, stiffness and pain of the neck, difficulty turning to the side; swollen, painful throat and submandibular region, this is quite abnormal, shoulders seem dislocated, upper arms seem broken, engendered disease: deafness and yellow eyes, pain in the lateral posterior aspect of the upper arm, elbow and forearm.

The Foot Tai Yang

- the bladder

The luo collateral

Excess: Nasal congestion with clear nasal discharge, headache, back pain.

Deficiency: Bloody nose.

The main channel

There can be rushes to the head, painful eyes, the nape of the neck feels tight and constrained, the spine is painful, the loins feel as if they are broken, the hips are unable to bend, the knee feels tied up, and the calf feels as if it were separated. There is a deficiency of qi at the ankle. *This channel controls the tendons* and gives rise to diseases such as piles, fevers, madness and insanity, pain in the top of the head and in the nape of the neck, yellow eyes, tearing and nosebleeds. There can be pain in the back, loins, buttocks, knees, calves and the feet. The little toe does not function.

Symptoms and conditions from the Da Cheng

Neck pain, pain in the eyes; nape, low back and leg pain, difficult to walk, dysentery, malaria, mania and withdrawal, heat in the heart and gallbladder; upper back arched, arms to the back, forehead and eyebrows ridged, nosebleeds, yellow eyes, contracted sinews and bones; prolapse of the rectum, hemorrhoids and fistulas, inflated abdomen and heart region.

The Foot Shao Yin

- the kidney

The luo collateral

Excess: Vexation and oppression, constipation and urinary block.

Deficiency: Lower back pain.

The main channel

One may feel hungry but does not desire to eat, the face is black like charcoal, there is blood from coughing or spitting, and there is a desire to arise when sitting. The eyes are blurred so that they are without perception. When the qi is insufficient, it results in fear. The heart is frightened and distressed. This is a deficiency in the bones. This channel controls the kidneys and gives rise to diseases where there is fever in the mouth, a dry tongue, a swollen throat, an upward flow of qi, the throat dry and sore, anxiety in the heart, pain in the heart, jaundice, diarrhea, pain in the spine, flaccidity, a fondness for lying down, and the bottom of the foot is hot and painful.

Symptoms and conditions from the Da Cheng

Black shanks on the legs, somnolence, no desire for food; the eyes are not bright, fever and mania, low back pain, leg pain, difficulty walking; the person acts like he is about to be captured, having difficulty hiding, heart and gallbladder trembling with fear, qi insufficiency; in addition, bound-up chest and yellow body.

The Hand Jue Yin

- the pericardium

The luo collateral

Excess: Heart pain.

Deficiency: Vexation in the heart.

The main channel

The palms of the hand may feel hot, the forearm and elbow being distorted and stiff, and there may be swelling in the armpit. In extreme cases there is fullness in the chest and ribs, and palpitations of the heart. The face can become red and the eyes may become a yellow color. There can be persistent laughter. This channel controls the blood channels and pulse, and may give rise to anxiety.

Symptoms and conditions from the Da Cheng

Hypertonicity of the hands; the arms are unable to extend, and are painful when they are bent; fullness of the chest, breasts and rib-sides, swollen axilla (unit) level; the heart is agitated and the facial complexion is red, yellow eyes, frequent laughter, cannot rest; heart vexation, heart pain, palms extremely hot.

The Hand Shao Yang

- the san jiao

The luo collateral

Excess: Spasms and cramps of the muscles around the elbow.

Deficiency: Atony of the elbows.

The main channel

Conditions can include deafness and tinnitus. There can be swelling and a sore throat. This channel controls the qi and may give rise to diseases where there is abnormal sweating. There can be pain at the lateral corner of the eye, at the cheek or jaw behind the ear, and in the shoulder and the upper limb. There can be a dysfunction of the ring finger.

Symptoms and conditions from the Da Cheng

When the three burners become diseased: deafness in the ears; throat impediment (bi), dry throat, swollen red eyes, pain behind the ears and in the elbows with sweating; pain travels between the spine and the back of the heart, wind is engendered in the shoulders and the upper back, radiating to the arm and elbows; incontinence (of urine) or dribbling blockage.

The Foot Shao Yang

- the gallbladder

The luo collateral

Excess: Inversion.

Deficiency: Weakness and atony of the lower limbs with inability to stand from a sitting position.

The main channel

There can be a bitter taste in the mouth and frequent belching. There can be pain in the heart and ribs, and the inability to turn or to lean. When extreme, it results in the face looking slightly ashen, the body being without oil and dry, and the lateral side of the foot being hot. This is from the Yang being deficient. *This channel controls the bones* and can cause diseases such as headache, and pain in the chin, jaw and lateral corner of the eyes. There can be swelling and pain in the center of the Broken Dish, swelling below the armpits, goiters under the arms, abnormal sweating caused by chills and fevers, and pains in the breast, ribs, buttocks and knees along the lateral surface of the fibula bone to the lower end and the area in front of the lateral malleolus and all the joints. The fourth toe may not function properly.

Symptoms and conditions from the Da Cheng

Pain of the chest and the rib-sides, the feet cannot be lifted, the face and body have no sheen, pain of the head and eyes; swelling of the supraclavicular fossa and axilla. Sweating like rain, goiter and tumors on the neck, hard like iron; malaria engendering cold and heat, connected to the bone and marrow.

The Foot Jue Yin

- the liver

THE LUO COLLATERAL

Excess: Swelling in the testicles, abnormal erection.

Deficiency: Sudden genital itching.

THE MAIN CHANNEL

There can be pain in the groin area, and one may not be able to bend down or look up. There can be hernias in men, and abdominal swellings in women. In extreme cases there can be a dry throat, an ashen face and a pale complexion. This channel controls the liver and may give rise to diseases such as fullness of the breast, vomiting, hiccups, diarrhea, recurrent hernia and weak or blocked urine.

SYMPTOMS AND CONDITIONS FROM THE DA CHENG

Scant qi and copious blood; males are dispersed and scattered, suffering low back pain; females have abdominal inflation, swelling of the lower abdomen; when it is severe: dry throat, the facial complexion is sloughing and dusty; engendered disease: chest fullness and vomiting; in the abdomen, diarrhea, and pain that does not stop, dribbling urinary blockage or incontinence of urine, shan (mounting), conglomerations and pain.

ENDNOTES

1. Ni, M. (1995) *The Yellow Emperor's Classic of Medicine: A New Translation of Neijing Suwen with Commentary.* Chapter 27. Boston, MA: Shambhala.
2. Ni, M. (1995) *The Yellow Emperor's Classic of Medicine: A New Translation of Neijing Suwen with Commentary.* Chapter 58. Boston, MA: Shambhala.
3. Wu, J. (2002) *Ling Shu or The Spiritual Pivot.* Chapter 10. Hawaii: University of Hawaii Press.
4. Wu, J. (2002) *Ling Shu or The Spiritual Pivot.* Chapter 10. Hawaii: University of Hawaii Press.
5. Wu, J. (2002) *Ling Shu or The Spiritual Pivot.* Chapter 10. Hawaii: University of Hawaii Press.
6. Wu, J. (2002) *Ling Shu or The Spiritual Pivot.* Chapter 10. Hawaii: University of Hawaii Press.
7. Wu, J. (2002) *Ling Shu or The Spiritual Pivot.* Chapter 10. Hawaii: University of Hawaii Press.
8. Ni, Y. (1996). *Navigating the Channels of Traditional Chinese Medicine.* San Diego, CA: Complementary Medicine Press.
9. Ni, M. (1995) *The Yellow Emperor's Classic of Medicine: A New Translation of Neijing Suwen with Commentary.* Chapter 56. Boston, MA: Shambhala.
10. Ni, M. (1995) *The Yellow Emperor's Classic of Medicine: A New Translation of Neijing Suwen with Commentary.* Chapter 58. Boston, MA: Shambhala.
11. Wu, J. (2002). *Ling Shu or The Spiritual Pivot.* Hawaii: University of Hawaii Press.
12. Wu, J. (2002) *Ling Shu or The Spiritual Pivot.* Chapter 10. Hawaii: University of Hawaii Press.
13. Wu, J. (2002) *Ling Shu or The Spiritual Pivot.* Chapter 10. Hawaii: University of Hawaii Press.

14. Wu, J. (2002) *Ling Shu or The Spiritual Pivot.* Chapter 10. Hawaii: University of Hawaii Press.

15. Wang, Z. and Wang, J. (2007) *Ling Shu Acupuncture.* Chapter 4. Irvine, CA: Ling Shu Press.

16. Yang, C. (2004) *A Systematic Classic of Acupuncture and Moxibustion.* Book II, Chapter 2. Boulder, CO: Blue Poppy Press.

17. Yang, C. (2004) *A Systematic Classic of Acupuncture and Moxibustion.* Book II, Chapter 2. Boulder, CO: Blue Poppy Press.

18. Wu, J. (2002) *Ling Shu or The Spiritual Pivot.* Chapter 10. Hawaii: University of Hawaii Press.

19. Wu, J. (2002) *Ling Shu or The Spiritual Pivot.* Chapter 10. Hawaii: University of Hawaii Press.

20. Wu, J. (2002) *Ling Shu or The Spiritual Pivot.* Chapter 54. Hawaii: University of Hawaii Press.

21. Ni, H.-C. (1979) *The Complete Works of Lao Tzu.* Chapter 25. Malibu, CA: The Shrine of the Eternal Breath of Tao.

22. Ni, M. (1995) *The Yellow Emperor's Classic of Medicine: A New Translation of Neijing Suwen with Commentary.* Chapter 5. Boston, MA: Shambhala.

23. Wu, J. (2002) *Ling Shu or The Spiritual Pivot.* Chapter 8. Hawaii: University of Hawaii Press.

24. Ni, H.-C. (1979) *The Complete Works of Lao Tzu.* Chapter 11. Malibu, CA: The Shrine of the Eternal Breath of Tao.

25. Wu, J. (2002) *Ling Shu or The Spiritual Pivot.* Chapter 71. Hawaii: University of Hawaii Press.

26. Ni, M. (1995) *The Yellow Emperor's Classic of Medicine: A New Translation of Neijing Suwen with Commentary.* Chapter 62. Boston, MA: Shambhala.

27. Lu, H. (1985) *A Complete Translation of The Yellow Emperor's Classic of Internal Medicine and the Difficult Classic.* Chapter 21 of the *Ling Shu.* Vancouver: Academy of Oriental Heritage.

28. Nghi, N.V., Tran, D., Viet, T. (2002) *Huang Di Nei Jing Ling Shu.* Chapter 21. Sugar Grove, NC: Jung Tao School of Classic Chinese Medicine.

29. Nghi, N.V., Tran, D., Viet, T. (2002) *Huang Di Nei Jing Ling Shu.* Chapter 21. Sugar Grove, NC: Jung Tao School of Classic Chinese Medicine.

30. Wilcox, L. (2010) *The Great Compendium of Acupuncture and Moxibustion.* Chapter V. Portland, OR: The Chinese Medicine Database.

31. Morant, G.S. de (1972 French edition, 1994 English edition) *Chinese Acupuncture.* Chapter V. Brookline, MA: Paradigm Publications.

32. Morant, G.S. de (1972 French edition, 1994 English edition) *Chinese Acupuncture.* Chapter V. Brookline, MA: Paradigm Publications.
33. Morant, G.S. de (1972 French edition, 1994 English edition) *Chinese Acupuncture.* Chapter V.Brookline, MA: Paradigm Publications.
34. Wu, J. (2002). *Ling Shu or The Spiritual Pivot.* Hawaii: University of Hawaii Press.
35. Wilcox, L. (2010) *The Great Compendium of Acupuncture and Moxibustion.* Chapter V. Portland, OR: The Chinese Medicine Database.

BIBLIOGRAPHY

Chamfrault, A. (1954) *Traité de Médecine Chinoise, Tome 1: Acupuncture, Moxas, Massages, Saignées.* Angoulême, France: Editions Coquemard.

Hudnut, F. (2002) *Surfing the Timeless Wave* (Vol. 1). Self-published: CreateSpace Publishing.

Lu, H. (1985) *A Complete Translation of The Yellow Emperor's Classic of Internal Medicine and the Difficult Classic.* Vancouver: Academy of Oriental Heritage.

Maciocia, G. (2006) *The Channels of Acupuncture: Clinical Use of the Secondary Channels and the Eight Extraordinary Vessels.* Oxford: Churchill Livingstone.

McCann, H. (2014) *Pricking the Vessels: Blood Letting Therapy in Chinese Medicine.* London: Jessica Kingsley Publishers.

Morant, G.S. de (1972 French edition, 1994 English edition) *Chinese Acupuncture.* Brookline, MA: Paradigm Publications.

Nghi, N.V., Tran, D. and Viet, T. (2002) *Huang Di Nei Jing Ling Shu.* Sugar Grove, NC: Jung Tao School of Classic Chinese Medicine.

Ni, H.-C. (1979) *The Complete Works of Lao Tzu.* Malibu, CA: The Shrine of the Eternal Breath of Tao.

Ni, M. (1995) *The Yellow Emperor's Classic of Medicine: A New Translation of Neijing Suwen with Commentary.* Boston, MA: Shambhala.

Ni, Y. (1996) *Navigating the Channels of Traditional Chinese Medicine.* San Diego, CA: Complementary Medicine Press.

Twicken, D. (2002) *Treasures of Tao.* Bloomington, IN: iUniverse.

Twicken, D. (2011) *I Ching Acupuncture—The Balance Method: Clinical Applications of the Ba Gua and I Ching.* London: Singing Dragon.

Twicken, D. (2013) *Eight Extraordinary Channels—Qi Jing Ba Mai: A Handbook for Clinical Practice and Nei Dan Inner Meditation.* London: Singing Dragon.

Twicken, D. (2014) *The Divergent Channels—Jing Bie: A Handbook for Clinical Practice and Five Shen Nei Dan Inner Meditation.* London: Singing Dragon.

Veith, I. (1966) *The Yellow Emperor's Classic of Internal Medicine.* Berkeley, CA: University of California Press.

Wang, Z. and Wang, J. (2007) *Ling Shu Acupuncture.* Irvine, CA: Ling Shu Press.

Wilcox, L. (2010) *The Great Compendium of Acupuncture and Moxibustion.* Portland, OR: The Chinese Medicine Database.

Wu, J. (2002) *Ling Shu or The Spiritual Pivot.* Hawaii: University of Hawaii Press.

Wu, N. and Wu, A. (2002) *Yellow Emperor's Canon of Internal Medicine.* Beijing: China Science Technology Press.

Yang, C. (2004) *A Systematic Classic of Acupuncture and Moxibustion.* Boulder, CO: Blue Poppy Press.

Yang, J. C. (2005) *Shen Disturbance: A Guideline for Psychiatry in Traditional Chinese Medicine.* Self-published.

INDEX

Printed and bound by CPI Group (UK) Ltd, Croydon, CR0 4YY
22/04/2026
02095185-0016